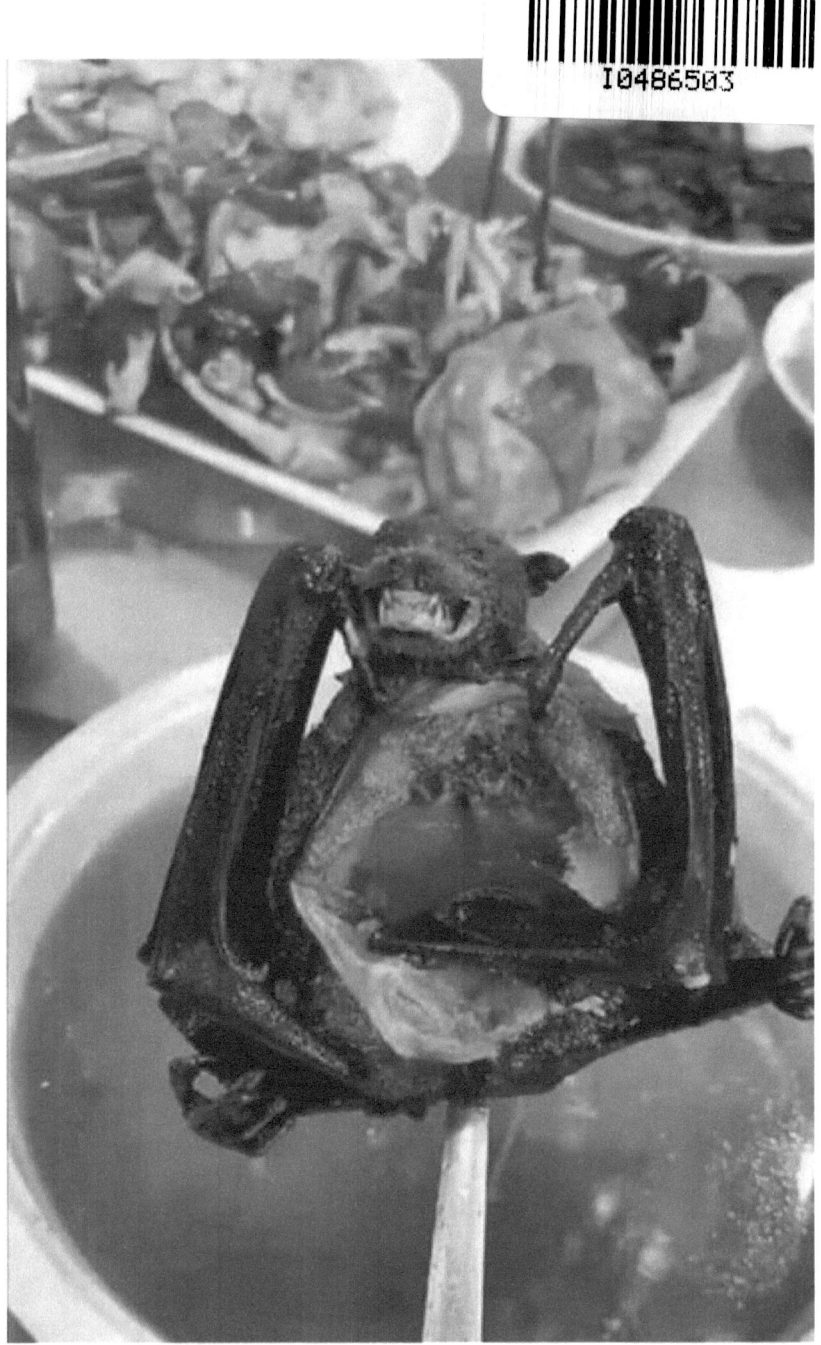

Bat soup

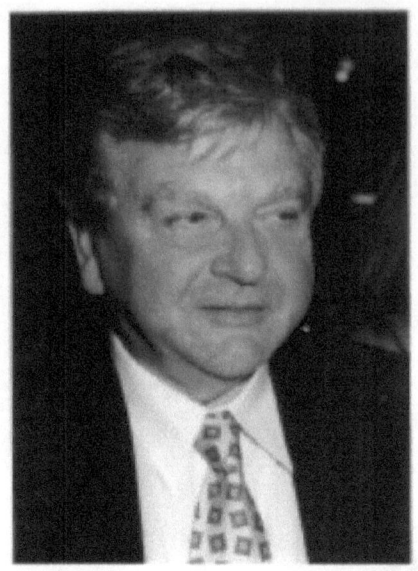

The Chinese Year of the Flying Rat, 2020 a BAT year

Paperback 158 pages Amazon.com ISBN 9798607753559
E-Pub Amazon.com

www.youtube.com [1]Peter Holst MD
www.preventingcancer.info[2]

1. http://www.youtube.com/

2.   http://www.preventingcancer.info

Gratitude

I would like to thank the Netherlands Prevention Fund for the financial support they have given to the research in my general practice, the research in collaboration with The Hague pulmonologists and the dust measurements by TNO in homes in Zoetermeer.

All research data were reviewed in collaboration with the statistical institute of the University of Leiden. This led to the publication at Springer Verlag of my book: Bird Keeping as a Source of Lung Cancer and Other Human Diseases. A Need for Higher Hygienic Standards. It was known that smoking cigarettes is bad for health but now it was shown that especially in bird breeders there is much more risk for lung cancer. This hobby is widespread in the Netherlands, Belgium and England, three countries with the highest lung cancer mortality rates in the world.

Despite the results of all follow-up studies, animal testing, serological research in new lung cancer patients in relation to breeding birds and keep pigeons, there is still no ban on imports of tropical birds in the much colder Western Europe. The number of smokers in the Netherlands has decreased with constant tax revenues. Asbestos remediation has been fully initiated, thanks to improved regulation of working conditions and environmental measures. In terms of size, the lung cancer problem due to the large-scale breeding of tropical birds and pigeons is even greater. It appears to be much more difficult to enforce regulation of the bird hobby. The bird unions react fiercely: take us first those cancer sticks of cigarettes before the government comes to our dear bird friends. My view is: breeding birds is fine, but do not lock them up in cages and leave them free and support nature conservation.

Foreword to the Original Studies

Original ideas and observations are rare. They are especially valuable if checked in practice, critically evaluated and supported by material independently collected by others.

It is to the very personal credit of Dr. P.A.J. Holst that he noticed a potential connection between the keeping of birds and the occurrence of lung cancer among members of households where they are kept. He has pursued the idea in his private practice and for over 12 years kept records of every single patient. The data were critically and statistically analyzed and supplemented by data and materials collected by lung specialists.

A new aspect is presented in this book. Avian products, spread in the house in the form of fine dust particles, may be inhaled deeply, cause irritation and contribute to local immune response in the lungs. It is hypothesized that this sequence of events is independent of other factors and significantly contributes to lung cancer and some other diseases.

It is a pleasure to work with a gifted man who is fascinated by many aspects of human wellbeing. The author is well aware of the importance of contact between mankind and nature. Living creatures such as dogs, cats, pet and aviary birds play a major role in human wellbeing. The keeping of birds may, however, as many other activities, also brings certain health risks. Holst analyses the habits of bird keepers and the consequences of bird keeping on the health of residents of houses where birds are kept. This book is a condensed presentation of an important scientific work contributing significantly to the health and well-being of mankind.

Professor P. Zwart DVM PhD
University of Utrecht, the Netherlands

Contents

Introduction

Since Aug 2018 there have been outbreaks of African swine fever in several provinces of China. At the end of 2018, the total amount of culled animals was 650,000. China's pig herd, by far the world's largest, was estimated then at 360 million animals. By the end of 2019, the number of pigs was half that of a year earlier, as an African Swine Fever epidemic spread to the world's largest pork producer. Up to 200 million pigs have been culled or died due to the disease, while pork output felt by 30%. Production may take more than 5 years to recover to previous levels before the deadly outbreaks as challenges including a lack of solutions to prevent the disease and a lack of capital will restrict restocking.

At the end of 2019, there was a first outbreak of corona virus in Wuhan, which has since been established to be the source of this virus. After the 2013 SARS epidemic, which spread from Hong Kong, Chinese virologists warned earlier that batborne CoVs will re-emerge to cause the next disease outbreak. China is a hot spot. Bats account for a quarter of mammalian species, rodents are 50 percent, and there's the rest of the mammals with us. Bats live on every continent, in proximity to humans, factory farms and life markets. The ability to fly of these flying rats makes them wide-ranging, which helps in spreading viruses, and their excreta can spread disease. Bats are host to a higher proportion of zoonoses than all other mammals.

Bats and rodents have been spreading diseases. Where rats and mice used to transmit diseases, nowadays the flying rats (bats) are the cause of this corona virus pandemic, originating from wildlife in life markets.

- **On February 24, 2020, the Chinese National People's Congress decided that illegal consumption and trade in wild animals will be "severely punished", as well as**

hunting, trade or transportation of wild animals for consumption.

- Stopping the sale of wildlife in markets is essential to limit future outbreaks of diseases that pass from animals to humans.

Human history on earth

We have learned by narration that paradise was located between Euphrates and Tigris. The first forms of life should rather be sought in the region of Great Pacific Ocean.

- 400 million years ago, Pan Gaia was surrounded by Pan Ocean.
- First, higher forms of life have evolved in Africa and have spread from there to the East and North.
- Great apes and large mammals did not exist in South America and Australia in prehistoric times.
- Finally, the Australian continent emerged from the Southland of the Pacific Ocean.

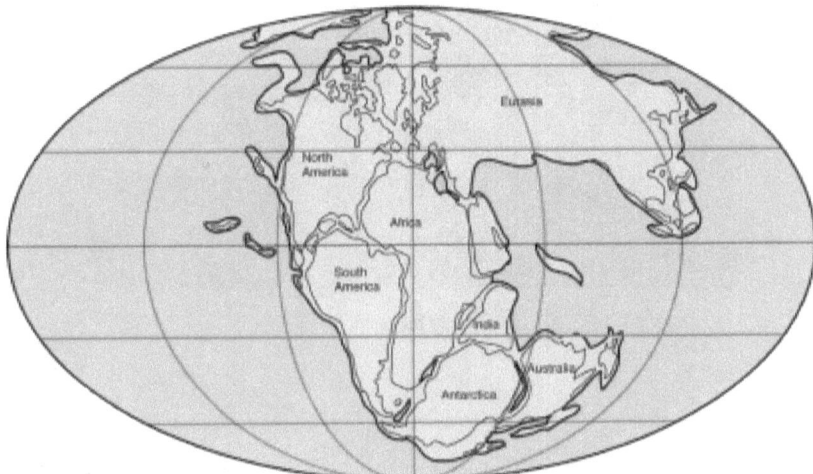

The first forms of life should be sought in the region of the Great Pacific Ocean. 400 million years ago, Pan Gaia is surrounded by Pan Ocean. The earth was a huge pancake. Life on earth has developed eastward under the influence of gravity, rotation of the earth and sunrise.

From Pan Ocean, the primordial soup, multicellular organisms, fish, marine iguanas and amphibians originated. Dinosaurs, birds, mammals and monkeys evolved on the land of Pan Gaia.

- Great apes, homo erectus and homo sapiens originated in central Africa and Asia.
- No great apes are found on the Galapagos Islands, Easter Island, Tahiti and other central Polynesian volcanic islands.
- North and South America were colonized from Asia not much earlier than 15,000 years ago.

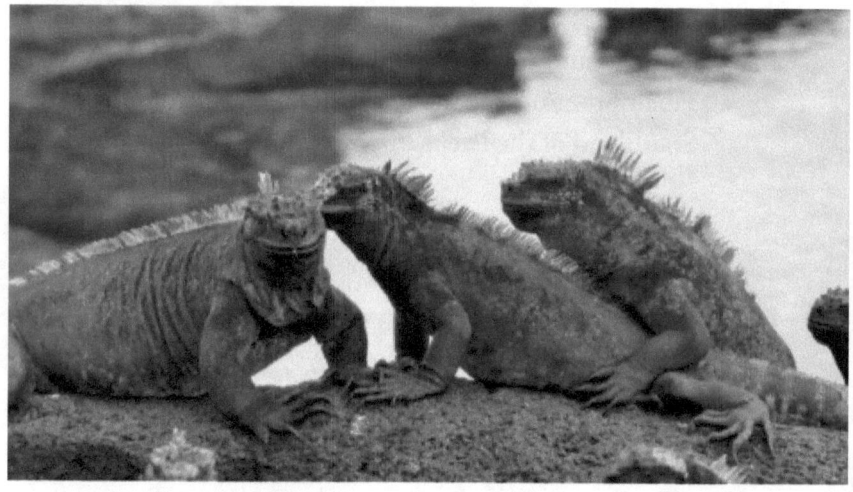

Marine Iguanas on Galapagos

Galapagos Islands

All first life forms live in perfect harmony side by side. The slaughter of turtles by corsairs and pirates has been a threat to the survival of this paradise on earth. Sea lions are the only mammals on these islands. Cattle breeding was later introduced on the Galapagos Islands and threatened to seriously disrupt this paradise. **50,000 goats must be killed, and all donkeys and domestic animals must be kept out of order to maintain this early original life**.

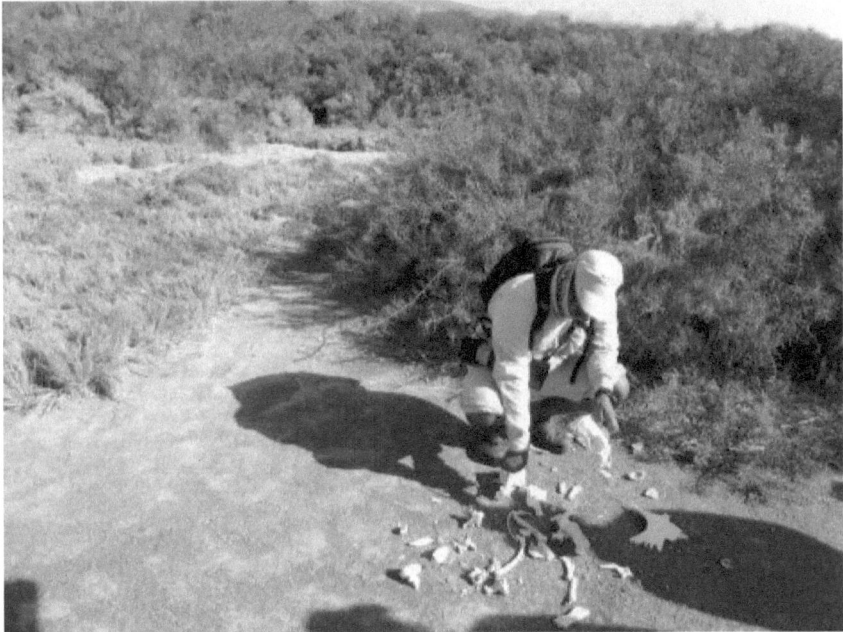

More than twenty percent of plant and animal species are found nowhere else in the world. Galapagos islands are the only place in the northern hemisphere where penguins live. Limited fish trade is allowed.

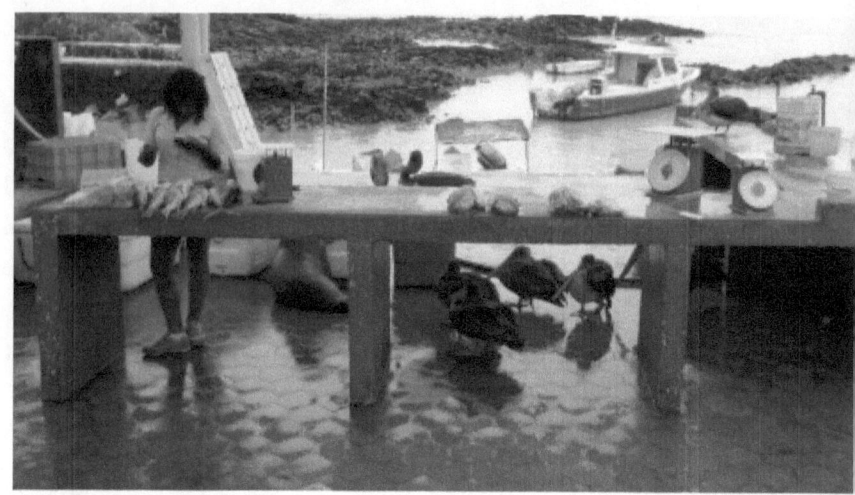

See this fish shop in Baltra, and how peaceful things work here

Farming on Galapagos, one of the world's most protected areas, is closely regulated. No heavy machinery, artificial fertilizers and pesticides are allowed. A fair trade in organic fruit and vegetables exists. In recent years chicken farms were introduced. There are now more than thirty intensive chicken farms on Galapagos, each rearing up to 4,000 birds for meat. Each of these farms rears a bigger population of individual chickens than the entire population of Galapagos penguins. In comparison with the tens of thousands of consumption animals in the chicken and pig farms of Western Europe, which are also fed with fishmeal and soya meal, this chicken breeding is very small-scale. Chickens in large numbers in confined conditions are more susceptible to affections like Newcastle disease virus and chicken leukemia virus. These viruses are a risk for the remaining penguins that have little immunity to novel diseases.

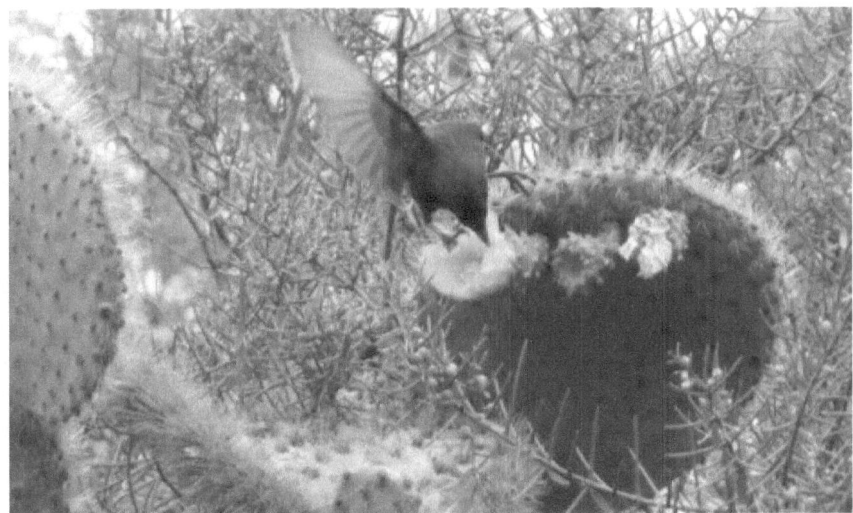

Finches on Galapagos developed under the influence of their environment

Darwin wondered after his comparative studies on the Galapagos Islands - The Origin of Species - what his findings meant for the further evolution of life on Earth.

- Charles Darwin showed that the finches on isolated Galapagos islands developed under the influence of their environment.
- **Darwin showed that environmental factors translate into physical and genetic characteristics.**

After his wanderings in the Malaysian Archipelago, Alfred Russel Wallace described the fundamental differences between the Asian part (Borneo, Java and Sumatra), separated by the Makassar Strait and the Australian part (New Guinea and Australia). The Asian continent with its great apes at the end of the evolution line borders here on the Australian continent that originated from tracts of land in the Southland of the Pacific Ocean. No apes were found on the Australian continent. Marsupials (kangaroo and koala) are the most developed life forms.

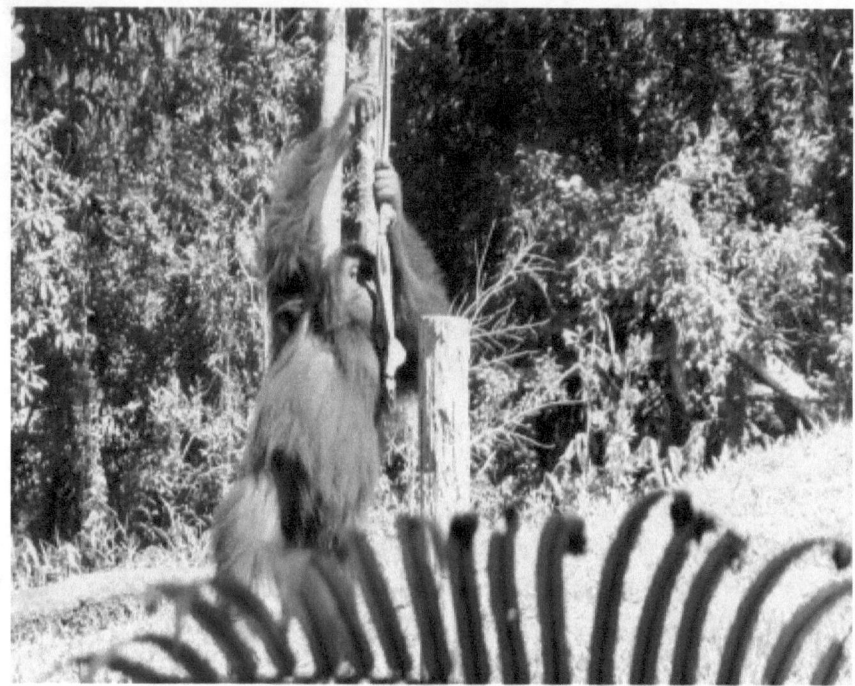

(*Alfred Russel Wallace*) *The Malay Archipelago, land of the Orangutan*

Of the branch on the heel. The orangutan has no tail and walk on two legs. Great apes have started to walk upright, on two legs. Standing, it is easier to gaze at prey or enemies, and arms that are not needed for locomotion remain free for other purposes, such as throwing stones or giving signals.

About a million years ago chimpanzees reached the warmer areas of Europe and Asia. From Africa through the Middle East, 60,000 years ago hominids reached Asia (*Homo luzonensis* and *floresiensis*) and 45.000 years ago Western Europe (*Homo neanderthalis*). People, chimpanzees and gorillas shared a common ancestor up to 5 million years ago.

All life is determined by double-stranded DNA or single-stranded RNA proteins. DNA is a wonderful self-regulating product. We share 85% of our DNA with chimpanzees.

- Watson and Crick have demonstrated the structure of the DNA with a double paired spiral staircase model. Acquisitions and characteristics of the ancestors are recorded in the stair steps.

In the mid-twentieth century, the sexual revolution took place with the invention of the contraceptive pill.

Homo sapiens has achieved greater dexterity in the East African region. From their tree huts in the tropical wood of Africa, the great apes developed a great hand skill. Man is the only man-like person who can place the thumb against the other fingers and make a precision grip with his hands. The more those hands were able to do, the more successful their owners were, so the evolutionary pressure led to an increasing concentration of nerves and extremely precise muscles in the thumb and fingers. The brain grew with it. As a result, people can perform particularly complex tasks with their hands. The sexual organs were at reach. Only modern man, due to the increased volume of the brain, has been able to control the reproductive processes and to free himself from the instinctive process of reproduction in the mid-twentieth century.

- **Factory farm animals are badly off with this new knowledge**

Artificial insemination techniques are also the result of this new insight. The increase in meat products and dairy production in the West could only be achieved with artificial insemination of mammals and the animals unilaterally fattening with soy flour, corn and fish meal.

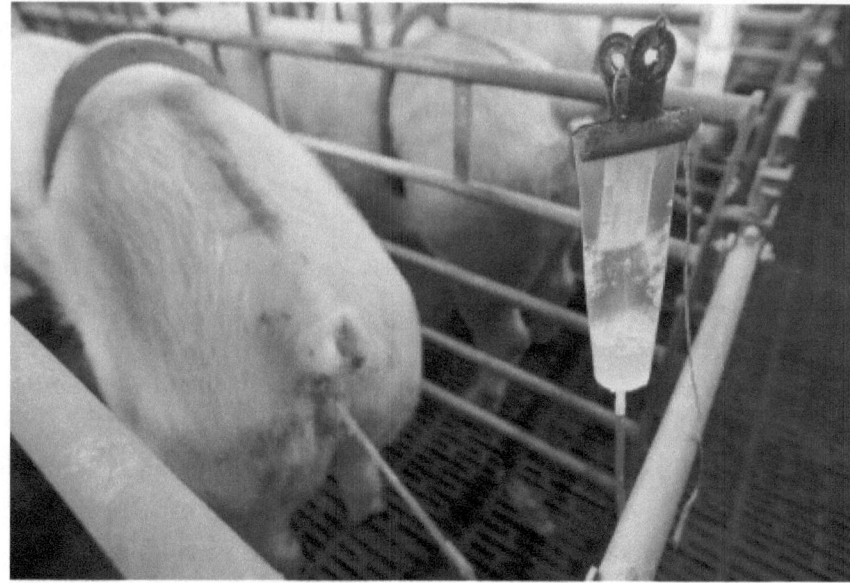

Artificial insemination of pigs in a factory farm
The unbridled breeding of animals, through artificial insemination of cattle and with incubators for poultry, has a devastating effect on our health, nature and the climate. Fast food, unnatural food and meat consumption lead to obesity, vitamin deficiencies, chronic diseases and premature death. Cancer is now the main cause of premature death.

The current stage in evolution

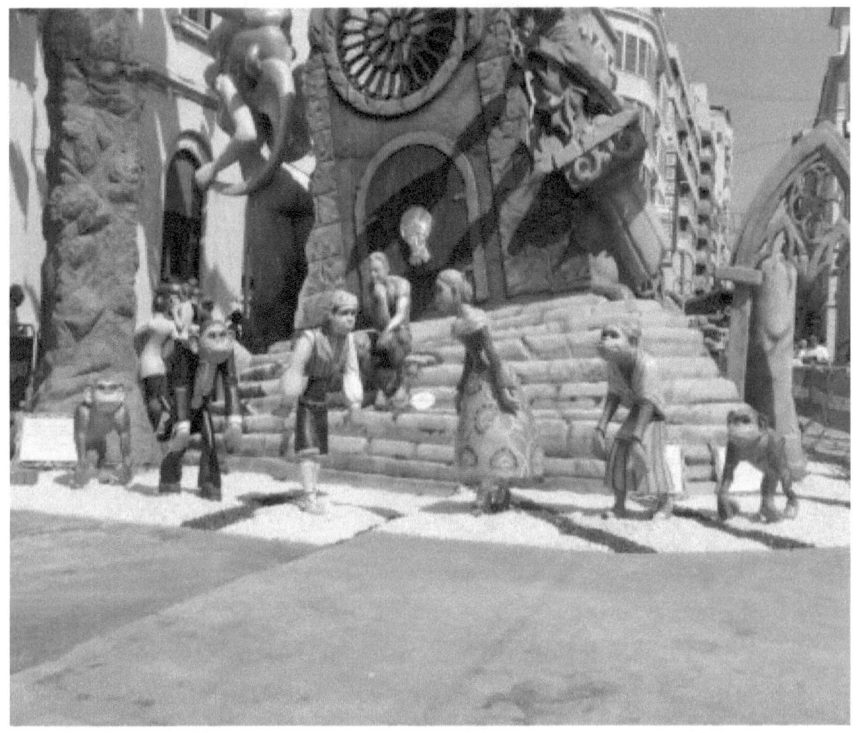

Man is the smartest because he got control over reproduction. Stick aging is still the highest attainable

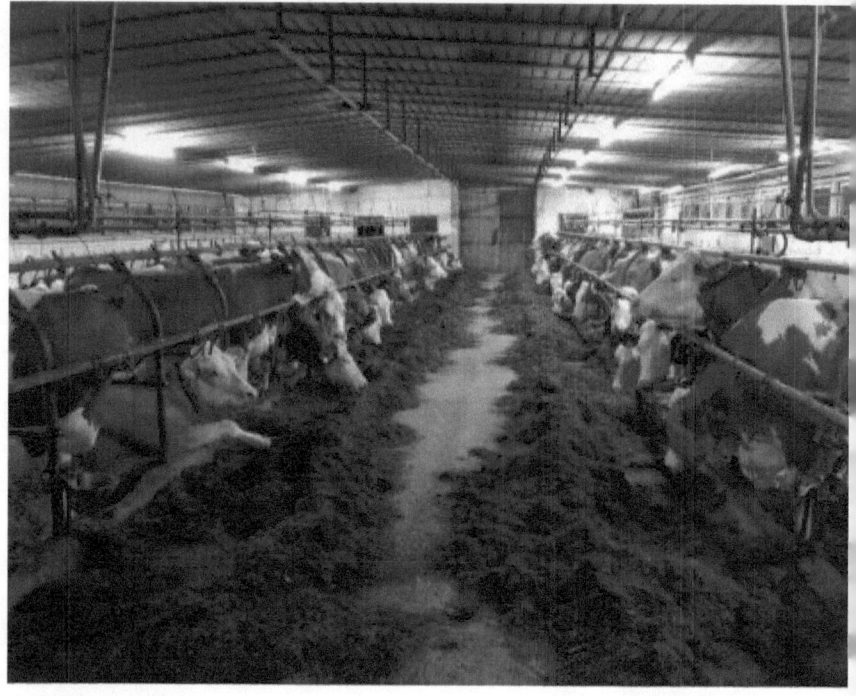

Factory farming

The downside of this control over reproduction is artificial insemination and factory farming of cattle. The cow must give birth to as many calves as possible for milk, cheese and meat. Calves were separated and grow up to be dairy cows, bulls go to the meat industry.

Sexuality in mammals

Most mammals have a tail, four legs, and their penis hangs on the lower abdomen. The great apes have no tail.

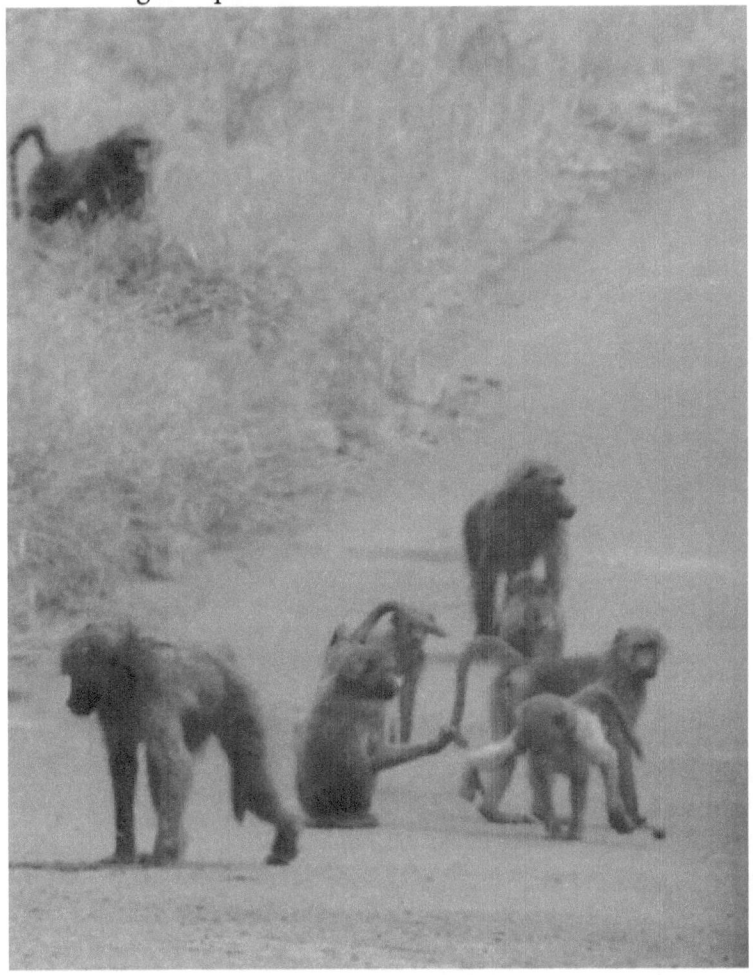

Receptive female monkey

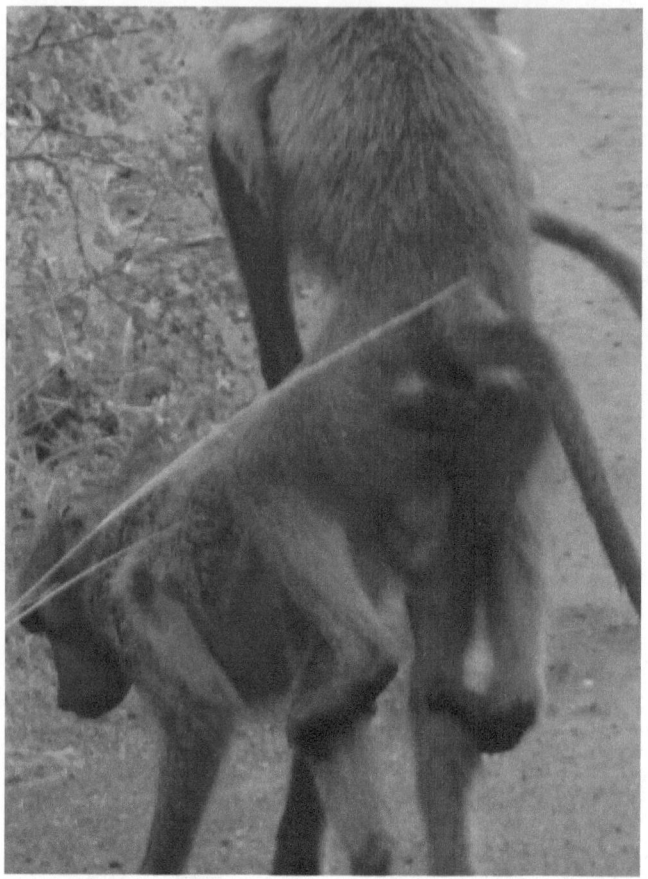

Monkey (baboons) and ape females advertise the time when they are ovulating. Their genitalia turn bright red, becoming receptive only at that time. They show their red badge of receptivity and proceed to have sex in public with any passing male.

In the earliest animal species the hormones released during orgasm induced ovulation. Mammals appear to be the first in which generation of ovulation has evolved. With 75 million years, spontaneous ovulation (and thus the menstrual cycle) is a recent development in the evolution of life on earth.

Although an egg is released roughly once a month in women, ovulation in some animals (such as rabbits) is triggered by having sex. According to Pavlicev and her team, hormones and brain pathways involved in such reflex ovulation could also be involved in causing a pleasant climax.

In 2016, the team analyzed 41 species of mammals. Fifteen of these species, including cats, koalas and camels, have reflex ovulation. The way these species are related indicates that this system was probably already present in the very first ancestors of mammals.

Evolution of spontaneous ovulation in mammals is correlated with increasing distance from the clitoris to the copulatory canal. With the evolution of spontaneous ovulation, orgasm was freed to gain secondary roles.

Pavlicev M, Wagner G. The Evolutionary Origin of Female Orgasm. J Exp Zool B Mol Dev Evol. 2016

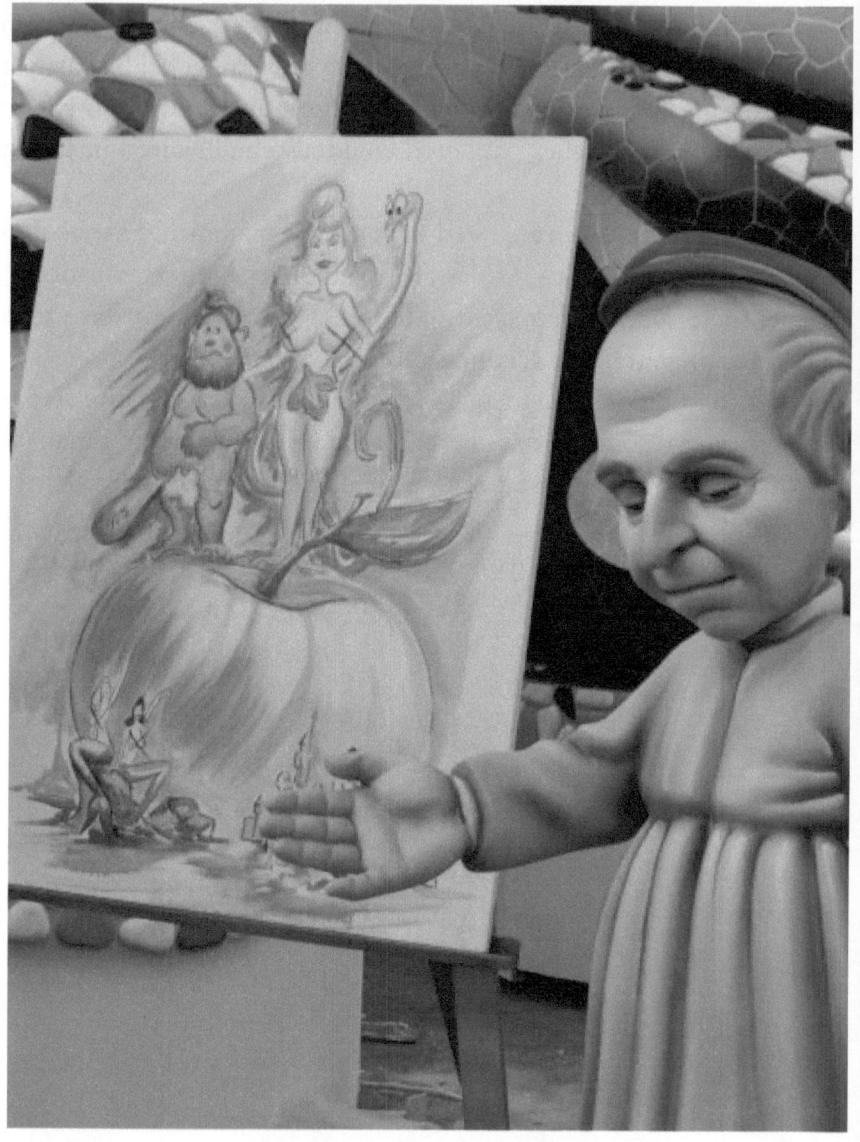

Because Adam and Eve had eaten the forbidden fruit in the Garden of Eden, man had lost his original perfection and eternal life

Contraception and religions

Man is banned from paradise and is doomed to multiply up tot the length of days and give birth to children. Later generations had inherited this imperfection and thus were in a state of sinfulness from birth. Because of that people could never get to heaven, but because of Christ's death on the cross, this original sin was taken away and it was possible for people who were baptized to look forward to a beautiful hereafter. (*Of course, people could just mess it up afterwards*)

Sexuality and Religion

Sacred eroticism. Before the beginning of the Roman era, in the seventh century BC, there were special temple priestesses whose job it was to keep the "Eternal flame" (symbol of the light of the Moon) burning. These women were known as the Virgins, not because they were celibate, but because they were not tied to a particular man. Virgin in the original sense therefore means independent woman and has nothing to do with prudency. The erotic rituals which these Virgins participated were dedicated to the Worship of the Mother Goddess. The symbol of the Mother Goddess was the Moon.

These women possessed a highly developed erotic energy that they could reflect in their profession. The difference with today prostitutes is that these women freely chose this profession and that they had the status of a priestess. What drove them was their love for their profession and their religious beliefs. The motive as not to succumb to manipulation, coercion or motifs that had something to do with money.

The ritual eroticism could lead to the birth of children. Such a child was seen as divine and not as illegal. That the father was not known, in the matriarchal culture prevailing at the time, was no problem. In the matriarchy, everything runs through the female line. In a patriarchal culture, it is important who is the father of a child.

When the patriarchal Romans took over the power in Italy, the rituals of these Virgins got another content. They were keepers of the eternal flame. However, the erotic rituals were banned. Furthermore, the patriarchal Romans saw the eternal flame mainly as a symbol of hearth and not as a symbol of erotic energy. Sex was forbidden. The Virgins were now called Amata (lovers), later Vestal Virgins. These were considered metaphorically as 'married' with the spirit of Rome. Famous Vestals from Roman mythology were Acca Larentia, Lupa and Rhea Silvia. In the same way, later celibate nuns were regarded as brides of Christ. The everlasting fire was extinguished in the fourth century DC by the emerging Christians, dealing with increasingly violent turn against other religions, and especially against an active role of women in religious life.

Heathendom and religions with many gods are characterized by erotic and fertility rituals. Polygamy is common. Monotheistic religions have strict regulations on sexuality and marriage. Monogamy is the rule.

The Christian Church

The early Christian view of sexuality gives the impression of being puritanical. Yet the Christian message to many in the classical culture was very appealing. Speaking of the early Christian church must be understood against the background of the ancient culture. In the first place, the classical culture was strongly layered. There was a big difference between free and slave. The life of a slave was not a pleasant life. In that world, Paul brings the message: "For as many of you as were baptized into Christ, have put on Christ. There is neither Jew nor Greek, the is neither bond nor free, there is neither male or female: for ye are all one in Jesus Christ. Everyone is equal before God. And in the church are no ranks or classes to apply. In that church, everyone is a brother or sister of another". A very remarkable thought in the classical world. In addition to this comes the powerful warning against all forms of sexual abuse and sexual violence are rejected. Sexuality should take place entirely on a voluntary basis and limited to the relationship of man and woman within their marriage. Various other forms of sexuality and violence are rejected. Strongly urges Paul to the monogamous marriage. Amidst all the humiliation and sexual violence that was given a new and original sound. Many in the classical world have also won for this message. The high moral standards that the early Christians stood for were a powerful propaganda for the Christian message. In the fifth century, including in Augustine, we see a radicalization of the Christian message occur. Augustine, who originally lived in concubinage, after his conversion to Christianity wanted a pure and chaste life. He thought it was better to have no sexual intercourse. The vision of Augustine has a strong platonic impact. The vision of Augustine's later celibacy formed celibacy for the clergy. This celibacy is still in force in the Roman Catholic Church. The Reformation has rejected celibacy for the clergy. Maarten Luther and John Calvin were married. All together it was the early Christian vision based on the ten Commandments, that sexuality was only allowed to get on a voluntary basis and in marriage between husband and wife. It was in the classical word a very remarkable message. This idea, however, was practiced by Christians with power. Celibacy was made an example. Sexual abstinence before marriage and for the clergy as a perpetual commitment were the logical consequence. As a reward eternal life.

The contraceptive pill since 1961

To put an end to the abuses in the Kempen that physician Ferdinand Peeters encountered in his daily practice, he went in search of a means by which the woman, for the sake of life, could arrange her own fertility. The contraceptive pill Enovid put on the market by the American biologist Gregory Pincus in 1957 still had too many side effects and was only admitted as a remedy for painful periods. In 1959, Dr. Peeters started a series of clinical tests with a hormone preparation offered by the German company Schering AG from his lab in the Sint-Elizabeth hospital in Turnhout. For six months, Dr. Peeters and his assistants Reimond Oeyen and Marcel Van Roy tested the preparation on fifty Kempen women for whom even more children posed a major health risk. After numerous experiments to find the right (more than half lower) dose of the two hormones (progestin and estrogen), in 1960 Peeters explained the findings to Schering in Berlin. The results were amazing. Not one of the women became pregnant and there were hardly any side effects. After Peeters' preparation (SH 639) was found to be safe and efficient in the United States, Japan and the United Kingdom as well, Schering markets the Anovlar pill in January 1961. Pincus tacitly acknowledged the superiority of Peeters' pill by halving the dose of Enovid in July 1961. In the end, it was Pincus who took the credit and (erroneously) went down in history all over the world as the inventor of the contraceptive pill. For fear of being robbed by the Church, however, the very Catholic Peeters did not give much publicity to his invention. Moreover, the pioneering research of a 'rural doctor' also aroused a lot of contempt among jealous professors from the KUL where Peeters was also active.

- For centuries, sheep intestine and since 1844 Goodyear rubber has been used as a contraceptive.
- The pill, IVF and artificial insemination brought the breakthrough in the middle of the twentieth century.
- The German company Schering AG put the Anovlar pill on the market in January 1961.
- The pill proved to be a particularly powerful emancipatory agent, both in America and in Europe. The pill radically changed the balance of power between men and women - and with it the entire society.
- By population control, the population growth decreased, while prosperity increased the dependency of the elderly decreased.

The Vatican

Proposed as a means to "regulate the fertility cycle of the woman through which periodic abstinence could be applied much more efficiently" in 1963, Peeters defended his invention during an audience with the then pope Pope John XXIII. In 1964 Peeters held a remarkable lecture with the same argument at the first congress of Catholic doctors in Malta. During the Second Vatican Council (1962-1965) Catholics were still fairly free and open about contraception. Peeters intervention did not fall on deaf ears because in 1965 the council reached a consensus with Gaudium et Spes. In it the council fathers wrote that the attainment of 'a generous but responsible fertility' is a matter between the spouses and God. This compromise was interpreted by some as the silent tolerance of the pill.

It all seemed so nice to start with the Second Vatican Council (1962-1965). The church opened its windows to the world and a fresh wind blew through the Roman Catholic Church. There was more attention for personal faith, reading the Bible and active participation in worship. In 1968, however, this back gate was closed again. Until Pope Paul VI published his encyclical "Humanae vitae", in which only in the (church-blessed) marriage there is room for sexual unification and reproduction. With this construction imposed by the Council of 1968, there was again a ban on contraception, even within marriage. The emancipation and changed role of women through education and labor participation will have alienated many from the church.

- Initially, a prescription from a doctor was required to start using the contraceptive pill.

- In the 21st century, the contraceptive pill is freely available at the drugstore.

- Even the morning after pill can be purchased at the drugstore and can be ordered online.

During a flight from the Philippines back to Rome in 2015, Pope Francis said that Catholics should not feel obliged to reproduce unlimited: "Some people believe - excuse the phrase - that to be good Catholics, they must be rabbits." he said regarding the prohibition of pill or condom in the Catholic Church. Francis speaks freely. But it would have been really revolutionary, if he had banned the outdated prohibition of birth control during marriage.

Hinduism and Buddhism

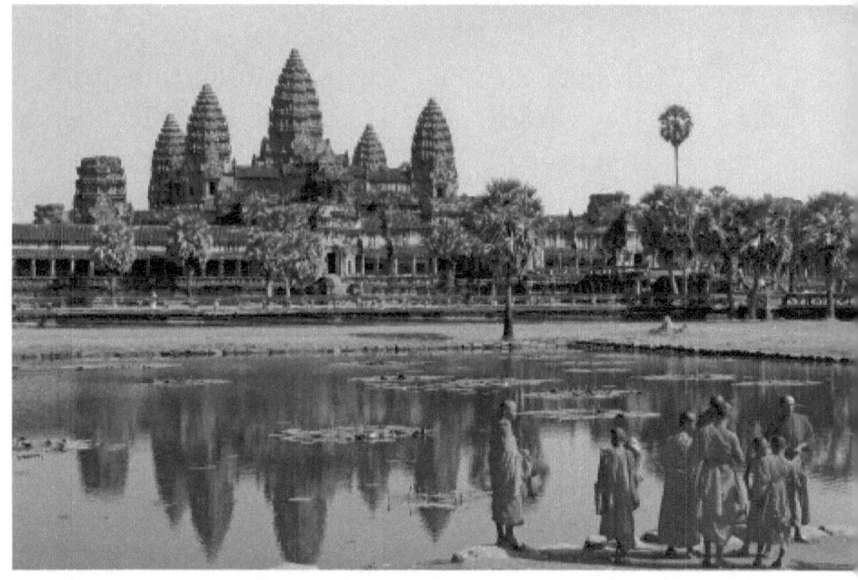

Angkor Wat in Cambodia is the largest religious building in the world, with an area of 1.6 km2. This temple city was designed and built in the early 12th century. By the end of the 12th century, Angkor Wat was transformed from a Hindu temple into a Buddhist temple, and has remained so until today. More than 100 religious buildings are spread over an area of 400 km2. The mysterious temples of Angkor are the remains of a disappeared civilization.

Buddha has forbidden erotic contact between monks and nuns. They must strive for liberation from the suffering of existence. A Hindu ascetic and the Buddhist monk and nun are highly appreciated in Asian cultures. By abstaining from sexual pleasures, they are outside earthly life and closer to the world of the gods. Because of the caste system, most Hindus do not marry the woman of their choice, but the woman who is arranged by the family. It is not uncommon for their marriage to feel trapped and the man or woman seek sexual pleasure outside of their marriage. The Hinduism and Buddhism are women-friendly philosophies of life. Whereas motherhood (Mary) is central to the Roman Catholic church, women are also seen as a lust object (Kamasutra) among Hindus and Buddhists. The Kamasutra, written by the philosopher Vātsyāyana in the third century, offers tips for the love life, such as finding a good wife, and how you can see if someone is interested in you.

Recently, the peaceful nature of Buddhism has been damaged. There are reports of sexual abuse, and the regimes in Buddhist countries such as Burma and Sri Lanka deal with religious minorities fairly harshly.

The Islam

Part of the Islamic culture is the pursuit of many descendants. In 2011 was predicted that the world's Muslim population will grow twice as fast non-Muslims over the next 20 years. By 2030, Muslims will make up more than a quarter of the global population. More than half of all Arabs are younger than 25. Arab societies have not enough sufficient economic and educational support for as many young people. Young families watch on television the lifestyle in the West and take over Western achievements.

Sharia law in Saudi Arabia and Iran:

- No freedom of religion or freedom of expression
- No democracy or a separation between religion and state politics
- No equality between people (the non-Muslim is not equal to the Muslim)
- No equal rights for men and women

There are many countries where the Sharia laws are fully applied. In Iran and Saudi Arabia, a woman is considered by law to be inferior to a man. Sharia courts in these countries ignore a woman's testimony if she does not have at least two men to support her testimony. In Iran, women are stoned on the basis of false accusations of adultery. In Saudi Arabia, women are beheaded in public. Penalties under Sharia law in Muslim countries are very barbaric and include stoning, amputation of limbs and execution for "moral" crimes.

The driving force behind Sharia and Muslim terrorism is the oppression of women. Strictly religious women surround themselves with a burka and are completely submissive to their husbands. Muslim suicide terrorists are promised that if they want to end their existence, a harem awaits them with virgin slaves.

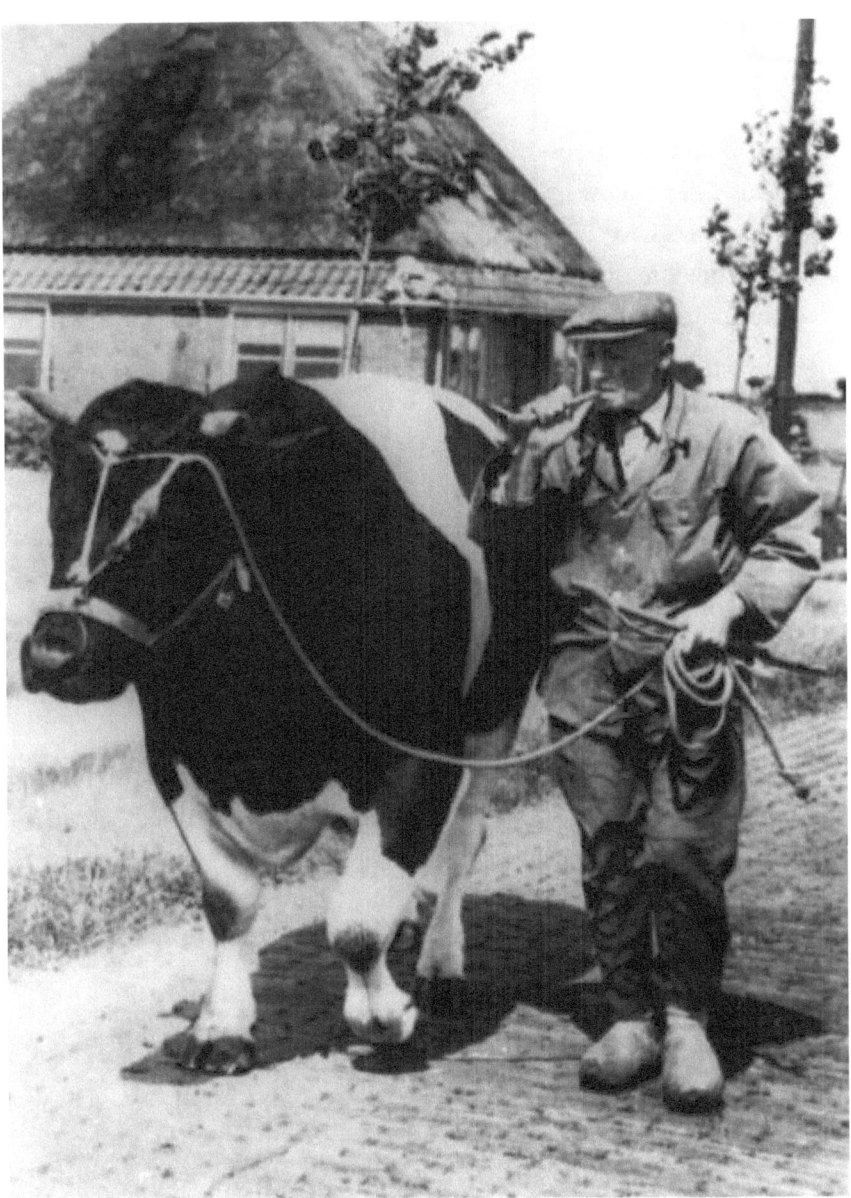

The bull runner went with the bull to farms where a cow had to be covered

Diseases from eating animals

Less than a hundred years ago the bull runner with the bull went to the farms where a cow had to be covered. Since the middle of the twentieth century we have a new situation, caused by intensive farming. All meat of farmed mammals is only produced by artificial insemination of cattle, pigs and rabbits. Mad cow disease, swine fever and bird flu are the result of intensive livestock farming.

Harmful consequences of artificial insemination of livestock

The population explosion and famine on earth have caused man to artificially inseminate animals and to breed exclusively for consumption. Fast food and an increase in meat consumption in the West are simulated in other parts of the world. Fast food, unnatural food and hamburger consumption lead to obesity and chronic diseases. In the meantime, the number of cancer diseases is increasing and is nowadays prime cause of chronic diseases and premature death in the elderly. The ceiling for meat and meat products has already been reached with the current 7 billion world population. The production of meat (products), poultry, pork and other meat tripled between 1980 and 2010 and is expected to double again in 2050

- **50 years of artificial insemination in mammals**

The increase in meat and dairy products is only achieved with artificial insemination of cattle. The production of milk, cheese and meat is inextricably linked. The cow must give birth to as many calves as possible for milk, cheese and meat. Female calves grow up to be dairy cows, bulls go to the meat industry. As a result, carcinogenic viruses are now found in cattle and in the meat and dairy industry. Harmful viruses such as Avian (poultry) leukemia virus (ALV) and Bovine (cattle) leukemia virus (BLV) are found in raw egg proteins and meat products. Harmful leukemia viruses from cattle and poultry

32

have spread to animal caretakers, employees in the meat and poultry industry and consumers (Johnson 2010, Blair 1982).

Global warming is largely the result of intensive livestock production. During the last ice age man was forced to eat more meat because there were fewer grains, fruits, nuts and seeds. Will modern man eat more vegetable food now that the earth is warming up?

The pig used to be kept as a food reserve for the cold winter months. Hams and sausages etc. We have started to eat more meat without fruit and vegetables. The theme of "artificial reproduction in mammals for increasing meat production" has never been brought before. Making livestock farming more sustainable is certainly not going to work to prevent global warming and the loss of plant and animal species. To make this book not only a message of doom I do proposals for more plant food and farming transition.

The farmers can repurpose their stalls with a power plant for heat and LED lighting. Strawberries, mushrooms, peppers, lettuce, grapes and pineapples can now also be produced in winter. With local production with a greater supply and diversity, the supply of fruit and vegetables over the equator will decrease.

Diseases in humans due to animal farming

Our dealings with mammals have been going on for thousands of years since we domesticated them. Infectious diseases that occur in animals mainly spread when large numbers of animals are brought together. A disease can then spread over the entire herd. Many farmers live close to their cattle and come into contact with their droppings, urine, breath, ulcers and blood. A disease can thus turn to humans and reach epidemic proportions if a group of people first come into contact with such a disease.

In the early Middle Ages (14th century) grain stocks of farmers in Mongolia attracted rats, marmots and mice. Rats and their fleas passed Pasteurella pestis (bubonic plague and lung plague) to the local population. The steppe marmot is the most common reservoir for

Pasteurella pestis in East Asia. The meat was eaten from the marmots and the skins were processed into fur. During the siege by the Mongols of the Genoese trading office Kaffa, on the Black Sea, hundreds of bodies of victims of the plague with catapults were shot in the besieged city to infect residents with plague. Genoese sailors were struck by the plague in 1345. Survivors and sick fled with their ships from the city to Sicily and Genoa. The Genoese fleet first contaminated the inhabitants of Messina in Sicily. From Genoa, the disease spread through the extensive trade network of Europe. The disease was spread throughout Europe.

- **The bubonic plague and lung plague killed 25 million people, 50% of the European population, in the 14th century.**

Cristobal Colon (Columbus) was born in Genoa, and more sailors from Genoa were undoubtedly signed on the ships of the explorers. They knew the history of this manner of warfare. In the conquest of South America, the Spaniards brought new diseases with them. Ironically, the only epidemic that Europeans brought back from South America was the syphilis, a not so enjoyable sexually transmitted disease.

- **Smallpox and tuberculosis have wiped out entire civilizations in South America in the 16th century.**

An Influenza A(vian) virus caused a flu epidemic in Fort Riley, Kansas. In this fort they bred chickens and pigs for the soldiers. A cook might have been infected with the virus. By mutation, the virus was able to bring about contagion from person to person.

- **The new bird flu virus (H1N1) was transferred by the troop transports in WW1 from the USA to Europe with** millions of deaths as a result.

Factory farming

The discovery of antibiotics and vaccines made it possible to keep cattle in large numbers. According to the BBC, the era of intensive livestock farming in Great Britain began in 1947. An agricultural law subsidized the farmers to stimulate production with new technology and to reduce Britain's dependence on meat imports. At the end of the last century, sheep heads containing prion particles from diseased animals were given to British cows. Natural herbivores - cows that eat grass and hay - were turned into carnivores, which ate meat and bone flour instead of grass, for faster growth and more financial gain. This caused the mad cow disease (BSE) due to damage to the brain and bones in the cow. The disease later also caused a variant of this in humans.

- **Mad cow disease (BSE) is spread by contaminated meat.**

Laying batteries

A study of 466 laying hens, ranging from 2 to 7 years, over a period of more than 3 years, has yielded data on reproductive organs and tumor formation in laying hens. Laying hens get ovarian cancer, but these tumors are rare in hens for the second year of life. At the commercial poultry farms, chickens are usually sacrificed after laying their first year, no later than 22-24 months old. Occasionally these hens reach a second leg year. Most cancers occur in these hens. The belly of the hens swells up due to fluid accumulation and the tumors are tangibly present. Of the 466 hens in this study, 149 (32%) developed ovarian tumors. The number of ovarian tumors was 39 (8%). In addition, 22 hens (5%) received benign swellings from the supporting tissue of the fallopian tube. In total, 45% of these laying hens received tumors from the reproductive organs.

- **Ovarian and ovarian cancer is most common in hens above the age at which most are slaughtered**

Chicken meat is highly contaminated

Every year, 45 billion chickens pass the world, along with 1 billion pigs, who can have contact with an estimated 50 billion waterfowl, such as ducks, geese and swans. Never before has the highly contagious avian flu, the influenza A avian flu virus, had such a chance to spread. Broiler chickens are bred to grow quickly in weight (Deshazo RD). In 1920 a chicken reached 1 kg in 16 weeks. The current broiler chickens now reach a weight of 2.6 kg, large enough for slaughter, in just 6 weeks. Over the past 50 years, growth has increased from 25 grams to 100 grams per day - an increase of more than 300%. Genetic selection is so intense that the age at which broilers reach their market weight and are slaughtered has dropped by as much as one day per year. Selection for rapid growth has resulted in poor health of the bones, causing deformities, lameness, tibia dyschondroplasia (TD) and ruptured tendons. Heavier broilers (> 2400 g) are often crippled. Sometimes the birds are no longer able to walk at all. Broilers and chicken products are heavily contaminated with antibiotic-insensitive (multiresistant) Escherichia Coli and are considered as a source of human infections. The percentage of infected chickens in Dutch broiler farms increased in the first week of life from 0-24% to 96-100%, regardless of the use of antibiotics and remained 100% up to slaughter (Dierikx CM). Multidrug-resistant intestinal bacteria were found in turkeys, cattle, chickens and retail meat products in Oklahoma. Sample were insensitive to commonly used antibiotics such as ampicillin, tetracycline, streptomycin, gentamycin and kanamycin. In Germany, multi-resistant staphylococci (MRSA) were detected in samples of turkey (40%) and broiler (25%). In pig farms too, with higher frequencies in fattening farms (73%) than in breeding farms (33%). Pork and chicken meat are potentially sources of multi-resistant species.

- **More antibiotics are provided to livestock than to humans.**

The increasing availability of antibiotics in the 1950s and 1960s was the reason to predict the 'beginning of the end' for infections. Nothing is further from the truth! Insensitivity to antibiotics increases and the arrival of new antibiotics decreases. Whatever the pharmaceutical industry is trying to do, there is no doubt that the microorganisms that have already existed for 3 billion years have adapted to survive under the most extreme conditions. Bloody diarrhea after eating insufficiently heated chicken or pork, for example after a barbecue, is a dangerous phenomenon. In some cases, bloody diarrhea is caused by multidrug-resistant Coli bacteria. Especially in women, these gut bacteria reach the bladder. The bacteria attach to the bladder wall and hardly respond to treatment with antibiotics. The urine becomes bloody. Not infrequently, these bacteria go higher and reach the kidneys through the ureter.

- **Entero Hemolytic E. Coli bacteria (EHEC) can cause severe kidney failure.**

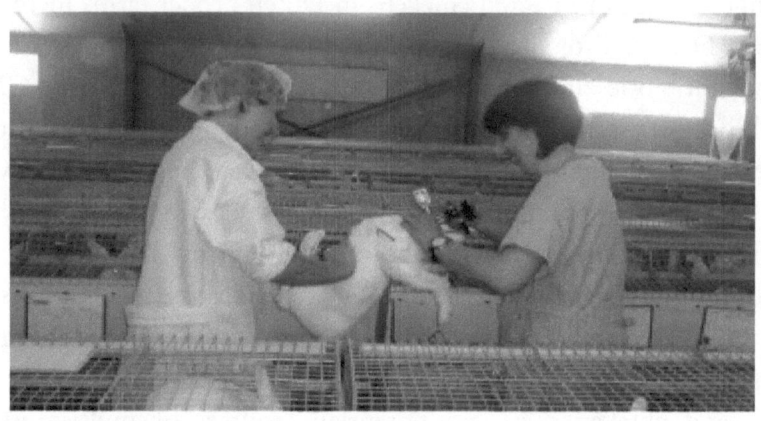

Rabbits are the second most bred animals in Europe

Female rabbits kept for breeding have specific problems. Those that are not used to feed the young are given little food and are often starved. On average, female rabbits are artificially inseminated 11 days after delivery. The impact of such a burden on their bodies is devastating, resulting in illness and death. More than 330 million rabbits are bred each year (more than all pigs and EU cows together). Every year more than a billion rabbits are slaughtered worldwide - most for their meat, a few for their fur. China accounts for about half that number, but the EU slaughters more than 326 million rabbits annually, especially in France, Spain and Italy. Most of them live in a small space. The majority is crammed in bare sheds with between 10,000 and 20,000 animals. The amount of space that is usually allowed for each rabbit is less than an A4 sheet of paper. While a well-groomed rabbit will live for about eight years or longer, rabbits reared for the meat are slaughtered at just three months of age. Of course, they can hop about 70 cm, but most commercially grown rabbits are not able to jump or sit up straight, instead of being able to jump. Because of the low height of their cages, some cannot even light their ears.

- **Hepatitis E virus (HEV) strains of reared rabbits indicate that these mammals can be a reservoir for HEVs that cause infection in humans.**

BBQ meat and hepatitis E virus

One in ten sausages and processed pork products in England and Wales can cause a hepatitis E virus (HEV) infection if the meat is not done, experts warn. Sausages must be cooked for 20 minutes at 70 degrees Celsius to kill the virus. There has been an "abrupt increase" in the number of cases in England and Wales, because people do not realize the risk. Hepatitis E is a liver infection that is spread by direct contact with fecal material from an infected person or by indirect fecal contamination of food or water sources. Pregnant women who become infected are at greater risk of acute liver failure, loss of the child and death.

Artificial Insemination

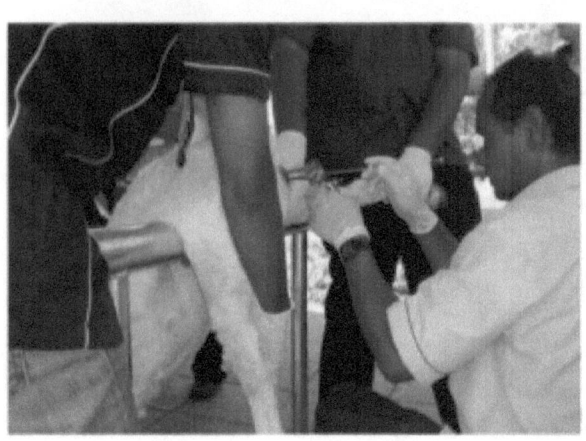

Intensive goat domestication and Q fever

Manure and straw from the goats are distributed by farmers as fertilization over the land. As a result, the Coxiella bacterium spreads through the air and infects the local population (Schimmer B).

Severe Acute Respiratory Syndrome (SARS)

SARS was caused by a corona virus and originated in South China province Guangdong (Canton) in November 2002. The worldwide outbreak of SARS was triggered on one day in a hotel in Hong Kong from a single person. A doctor from Guangdong participated in a grand wedding party. When the guests left, the virus, coughed up by this doctor, spread to five countries within 24 hours. In a few months, this coronavirus spread to 30 countries on six continents, producing 8,096 probable cases and 774 deaths (WHO 2004). In the past a trip around the world took a year; today, we with our viral luggage can travel around the earth in 24 hours. The Guangdong authorities cleared thousands of civet cats and other wild animals in January 2004. They also imposed a permanent ban on the trade and human consumption of civet cats. Researchers showed that humans and civet cats had viruses with the same genetic profile, after testing six SARS-carrying civet cats from a restaurant. At the beginning of 2004, a waitress was infected by the SARS virus. WHO experts also demonstrated the virus in cages of a restaurant where a SARS patient had eaten meat from civet cats. Unfortunately, Chinese people prefer a large range of wild animals, and the civet cat is considered a delicacy in South China. In rural China, the animals are still sold on the markets.

Dromedary flu (MERS-Corona Virus)

Dromedary flu, from virus-spreading young camels, is the result of intensive camel breeding on the Arabian Peninsula. There is a rapid increase in the number of reported infections with Middle East Respiratory Syndrome Corona Virus (RNA virus). Since June 2012, MERS-CoV has infected more than 1,814 people, including 734 deaths (41%). The disease first appeared on the Arabian Peninsula, in Saudi Arabia and the United Arab Emirates. Concerns about the situation have increased considerable, particularly concerns about the spread of the infection in hospitals and in contacts with patients. Dromedary flu is endemic among young camels in Saudi Arabia. Sick camels separate corona viruses from their noses and sometimes in the stool. Only recently people and dromedary camels share the same corona viruses. The corona virus first adapted in the herds of camel breeders, especially in newborn camels. Young camels are more susceptible to the corona virus, because of their lower immunity status and the smoother virus replication. Dromedaries bred as dairy cattle (females) showing highest serum titers, followed by camels being bred for meat (mostly males) and finally the dromedaries used for transport activities (also mostly males) have been found to be the least susceptible to the virus. Young camels that do not have antibodies have a high chance of becoming infected and, in turn, expose the mothers to infection or reinfection. Camels are also bred in Burkina Faso, Ethiopia and Morocco under the same conditions. Today the MERS-CoV circulates from person to person. Corona viruses adapted to humans spread through the airways and circulate more and more in society. With the annual Hajj pilgrimage to Mecca, more than 2 million Muslims, from more than 180 countries, are at risk of becoming infected with MERS-CoV and spreading. Saudi authorities warn not to drink unpasteurized camel milk and to wear gloves when caring for the animals. The omnipresence of the animals, their importance for the economy of the regions and their popularity will continue to promote the transfer of this coronavirus from dromedary to human.'

The slaughter of chimpanzees, cause of global spread of AIDS

HIV/AIDS spread to humans through human consumption of meat of wild animals (chimpanzee and gorilla) in Central Africa. During the 20th century, commercial hunting using firearms and wire snares to supply lodging and oil exploration operation concessions along new roadway networks has dramatically increased the catch in Central African forests. Annually, it is estimated that 579 million wild animals are caught and consumed in the Congo basin, equaling 4.5 million tons of bush meat.

The year the global eradication of smallpox was declared (WHO 1980), the first reported cases of AIDS were being identified. Since then, HIV/AIDS has resulted in an estimated 65 million infections and 25 million deaths. In several African countries, the estimated prevalence of HIV now exceeds 20% of the adult population. Although blood banking, the relaxation of sexual mores, and injection drug use facilitated the spread of HIV, the simplest and most plausible explanation for the emergence of the virus appears to be exposure to animal blood or excretions as a result of hunting and butchering primates, or the subsequent consumption of uncooked or contaminated bushmeat. **Blood samples obtained from 573 freshly butchered primates in logging concessions and bushmeat markets** found 18.4% with evidence of Simian Immunodeficiency Virus (SIV), considered the precursor to HIV. Although HIV-like viruses have been recently discovered in gorillas, the butchering of chimpanzees is considered the most likely source for HIV-1, the strain of the AIDS virus that has spread around the world. Molecular analyses now suggest SIV crossed species not once, but on no fewer than eight separate occasions in recent history. Until a few decades ago, such a zoonotic transmission event may have only affected a small number of isolated rural villages. Corporate logging for export expanded western Africa's tradition of primate subsistence hunting into a major commercial enterprise that extends into surrounding major cities where ape meat garners premium prices in restaurants. By the frequent rotation of sex workers into logging camps of timber companies, the routes of transmission along roads cut by deforestation in Africa run in both directions. In addition to concurrent socioeconomic disruptions of postcolonial, sub-Saharan African infrastructure, widespread iatrogenic and self-injection use of unsterile needles may have played a role in the cross-species adaptation of the virus and account in part for the simultaneous appearance of multiple strains of HIV across Africa. Similar possible iatrogenic facilitation of infection has been reported with parenteral, antischistosomal vaccination in Egypt, which may have led to widespread hepatitis C virus distribution, as well as the exposure of millions of Americans to simian virus 40 in batches of polio vaccine between 1955 and 1963. For most zoonoses, humans are the deadend host. In terms of global public health implications, the greatest concern surrounds zoonotic infections like HIV/AIDS that can not only jump from animals to humans, but can then spread human-to-human. More people engage in sexual activity than the butchering of chimpanzees. Emerging retroviruses are of special concern because of their ability to integrate into the DNA of the host cell. Making their copies is done with the enzyme reverse transcriptase that is already in the virus, often with the necessary copying errors. As a result, it has not been possible to develop a good vaccine against HIV/ AIDS. There are seven genera in the Retroviridae family: lentivirus, including HIV and SIV, spumavirus, and five groups of cancer-causing retroviruses previously clustered together as oncovirus. SIV is just one of a large reservoir of poorly characterized lentiviruses in African primates raising the specter of additional AIDS-like zoonoses arising from continued bushmeat consumption. The Ebola virus is one of those.

Bushmeat, cause spread Ebola

Ebola is believed to be spread over long distances by bats, which can host the virus without dying, as it infects other animals it shares trees with such as monkeys. It often spreads to humans via infected bushmeat. Ebola virus is the cause of one of humanity's deadliest infections, but is not efficiently spread compared to a virus like HIV. Ebola seems to begin when hunters kill infected animals and eat the meat poorly cooked or even merely touch the meat as they bring it to market and/or prepare it. Hunters find dead animals in the jungle and also bring to the market the flesh of chimpanzees and gorillas died of Ebola. The droppings of infected animals on edible vegetation are also a source of infection. The animals most pointed to as carriers of Ebola virus are various species of fruit bats. These often large bats are frequently dried and then eaten directly or made into soup. It is estimated that each year 28,000 fruit-eating bats, worth € 6 each, annually are sold in Ghana. The fruit-eating bats are reservoirs of the virus, but not harmed by it. Other animals harbor the virus too. Some are sickened and killed by it such as the great apes and pigs, but they infect other apes and humans. Other animals too are probably reservoirs. Once a person has contacted the disease, the virus readily spreads without further spillover from infected animals. The profuse bleeding and expulsion of other bodily fluids from infected people, often spreads the infection to a large number of those who touch the patients, their clothing, or fluids. The Ebola virus is transmitted among humans through close and direct physical contact with infected bodily fluids, the most infectious being blood, faeces and vomit. The Ebola virus can also be transmitted indirectly, by contact with previously contaminated surfaces and objects. The risk of transmission from these surfaces is low and can be reduced even further by appropriate cleaning and disinfection procedures.

There is a new epidemic every few years since 1976. The seventh Ebola virus outbreak began on July 26, 2014 in the Democratic Republic of Congo (DCR). A pregnant woman was infected by her husband who brought contaminated meat. She fell ill on July 26 and died August 11. A local doctor and three assistants performing a post-mortem caesarean section (to separate the fetus from the mother for funeral, according to local culture) also became infected and died. These health workers were the source of further cases of this epidemic.

Maganga GD (2014) Ebola virus disease in the Democratic Republic of Congo (DCR).

New England Journal Medicine.

A tenth Ebola outbreak began on August 1, 2018 in Mangina DCR and caused 3,444 illnesses until March 2020, of which 2,264 deaths

The hunt for bushmeat is the greatest threat to great apes. Due to small populations and their slow reproduction, apes are very vulnerable. Contact between humans and apes creates a risk of spread of diseases with them. Ebola is particularly deadly. Since 1990, a total of as many as a third of gorillas that live in national parks and other protected areas, deceased from this disease.

Wuhan Acute Respiratory Syndrome (COVID-19)

Since the end of 2019 a new coronavirus epidemic has been spreading from the Chinese metropolis of Wuhan. A blood test has enabled labaratories to charactarize this RNAvirus and to monitor the spread of the virus in new patients. One third of the patients enter the ventilation unit of the intensive care with deep pneumonia, not bronchitis but pneumonitis. This resulted in a life-threatening decrease in lung capacity. It has been shown that the first patients with pneumonia appeared at the Wuhan live market where exotic animals as snakes, turtles, bats, foxes and porcupines are sold for consumption. Even civets, a cat-like creature, were still among dozens of species listed on an exhaustive price list for one of the animal trading businesses at the Wuhan market. The first studies indicate that horseshoe bats or fruit bats have spread the virus to snakes and rats. The animals are locked up in small cages day and night for days and it is not inconceivable that bats, also known as the flying rats, infected them or their food with the coronavirus. Live markets in China are held responsible for the outbreak of the SARSvirus in 2003 with more than 6.000 confirmed cases and that killed more than 800 people worldwide. At 26 Jan 2020 COVID-19 caused 2751 confirmed infections with 56 deaths in China since the beginning of January, and spread to about a dozen countries. At 31 Jan there were already more than 9700 confirmed infections in China, with 213 deaths. Already more cases than the total of the SARS epidemic. On March 4 there were 80,409 registered cases with 3285 deaths and a spread to 86 countries

Bat coronaviruses also caused SARS and MERS epidemics and a highly destructive epidemic in pigs. Bats are the only flying mammals, they devour disease-carrying insects by the ton, and they are essential in the pollination of many fruits, like bananas, avocados and mangoes. They are also an incredible diverse group, making up about a quarter of all mammalian species. Their ability to coexist with viruses that can spill over to other mammals, in particular humans, can have devastating consequences when we eat them, trade them in livestock markets, and invade their territory. Certainly, rodents, primates, and birds as psittacines and doves also carry diseases that can jump and have jumped to people: bats are far from alone in that regard. In the contrary bats are more numerous and widespread. While bats account for a quarter of mammalian species, rodents are 50 percent, and then there's the rest of us. Bats live on every continent exept Antarctica, in proximity to humans and farms. The ability to fly makes them wide-ranging, which helps in spreading viruses, and their feces and urine can spread diseases. Bats often live in huge colonies in caves, where crowded conditions are ideal for passing viruses to one another.

Employee risks in the meat industry

An increased mortality of brain tumors has been observed in veterinary surgeons (Blair A). Veterinarians and Artificial Insemination assistants do a lot of internal research on cows. Transmission via the uterus and the birth canal during labor, of bovine leukemia virus (BLV) plays a crucial role in the spread and persistence of BLV infection in cattle (Mekata H).

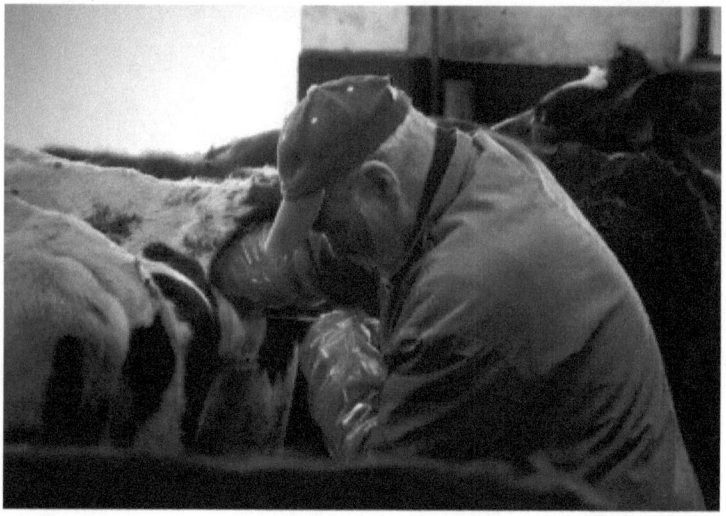

In their work, veterinarians and AI staff come into contact with bovine leukemia virus (BLV), a carcinogenic virus. Bovine leukemia is an economically important infection of dairy cattle worldwide. The presence of infections in Canadian dairy herds is high and is still increasing. Seventy percent of the herds were identified as BLV positive (one or more positive animals).

Nekouei O, VanLeeuwen J, Sanchez J, Kelton D, Tiwari A, Keefe G Herd-level risk factors for infection with bovine leukemia virus in Canadian dairy herds. Prev Vet Med. 2015; 119 (3-4)

The deaths of 5,016 veterinarians were examined and compared with those of the general American population. The mortality rates were significantly increased from malignant lymphomas and leukemia, colon, brain and skin. Less mortality was found for stomach and lung cancer.

Blair A, Hayes HM Jr. (1982) Mortality patterns among US veterinarians, 1947-1977: an expanded study. Int J Epidemiol. 1982 Dec;11(4):391-7.

Increased risk of esophageal, colon, brain and pancreatic cancer and melanoma in veterinarians in Sweden could not be explained by the socio-economic status of this profession. Occupational exposures to carcinogenic viruses in livestock are potential sources.

Travier N, Gridley G, Blair A, Dosemeci M, Boffetta P. (2003) Cancer incidence among male Swedish veterinarians and other workers of the veterinary industry: a record-linkage study. Cancer Causes Control. 2003 (6):587-93.

Cows are constantly re-impregnated after the birth of the calves by artificial insemination, so that their milk will never stop flowing. The sperm is frozen in "straws" and then introduced by a veterinarian or AI assistant to the animal at the right time, depending on the time of the ovulation cycle. Calves are taken away from their mother soon after birth. Their calves grow up to become dairy cows or are reared for veal. For production of milk and cheese, the mother cow must give birth to as many calves as possible. Female calves grow up to become dairy cows, bulls go to the meat industry. Milk, cheese and meat production are inextricably linked.

Why people have become carnivores

The slaughtering of animals is a result of our ancestors' struggle against wild animals, lions, elephants, bears etc.

From Africa and the Middle East, homo sapiens reached Western Europe 45,000 years ago.

- In that period, lions and other predators were still in the majority
- Neanderthals were the first to make the art of fire in Europe
- With wooden arrows and stone axes, there was control over lions, bears and other wild predators
- Modern man has gotten smaller jaws and larger brain contents than the Neanderthals by cooking and roasting meat

In the Colosseum, fighting of humans against wild animals took place until the 6th century. In bullfights, such as in modern corridas, bulls were hunted by helpers until they became angry: the toreros, the real hunters, fought the bull on foot, with a club or a lance. Other bullfights were related to skills similar to those depicted on famous Cretan photographs or contemporary rodeos: unarmed men on horseback rode on the bull to defeat him and then jumped on the bull to throw him down and turn his neck.

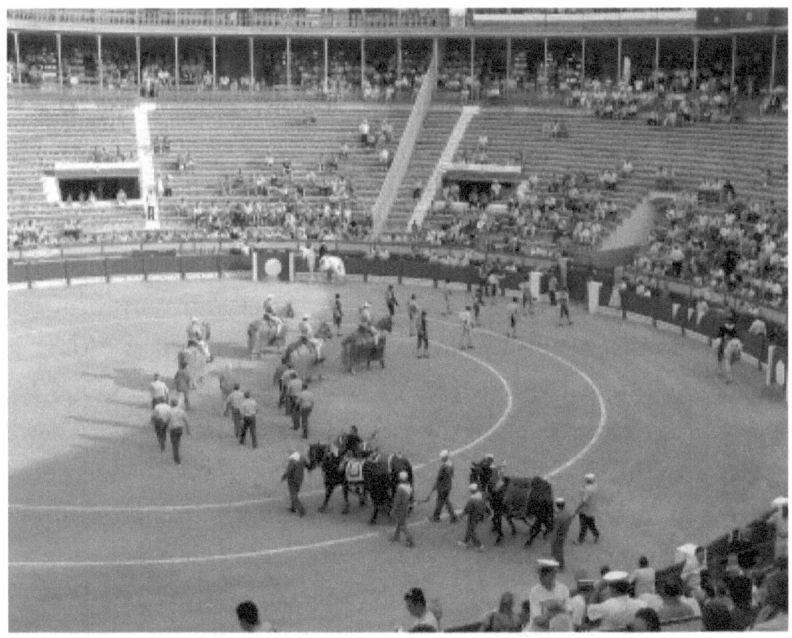

Parade of a bullfight (Plaza de Toros, Alicante)

- Bullfighters walk in front

- The helpers follow

- Picadores on horseback

- Animal handlers

- Cleanup team for killed bulls

- Butchers close the procession

Employee risks in the poultry industry

Carcinogenic viruses are found and cause tumors in chickens and turkeys. A number are carriers and diffusers of these infectious viruses. Virus has been shown in chicken products and eggs, so exposure to humans is universal and almost unavoidable. These viruses are not very contagious, but still have the ability to infect and transform human cells. Antibodies against avian leukemia sarcoma viruses (ALSV) and reticulo endothelial viruses (REV) have been found in blood sera of workers in poultry slaughterhouses. Mortality from cancer has been studied in 20,132 workers in poultry slaughterhouses and processing plants, a group with the highest human exposure to these viruses. The mortality rate among poultry workers has been compared with that of the American population as a whole. Substantially increased risks were observed in poultry workers as a whole or in subgroups, for different cancers: cancer of the mouth and pharynx; pancreas; trachea / bronchus / lung; brain; cervix; lymphocytic leukemia; monocytic leukemia; and tumors of the blood-forming and lymphatic systems. This study provides evidence that a group of people with high exposure to carcinogenic viruses, occurring in poultry, are at a higher risk of death from a number of cancers. Antibodies have been shown in the blood of these workers against avian leukemia viruses (ALV) and reticulo endothelial viruses (REV).

Metayer C, Johnson ES, Rice JC (1998) Nested case-control study of tumors of the hemopoietic and lymphatic systems among workers in the meat industry. Am J Epidemiol 147(8):727-38 https://www.ncbi.nlm.nih.gov/pubmed/9554414

Johnson ES, Ndetan H, Lo KM (2010) Cancer mortality in poultry slaughtering / processing plant workers belonging a union pension fund. Environ Res 110(6):588-94 https://www.ncbi.nlm.nih.gov/pubmed/20541185

Brain cancer is more common in poultry farmers involved in killing chickens. The killing of chickens was accompanied by an almost 6-fold increase in the risk of brain cancer. Workers in poultry slaughterhouses and processing plants often process thousands of chickens daily, come into contact with poultry meat, organs and blood and run the risk of injuries that form a route for viruses and other microbial substances to enter the body. They also work for longer periods in confined spaces, which increases the risk of inhaling microbes. Viruses that are known to cause cancer in poultry can be responsible for the increased incidence of cancer in poultry farmers killing chickens.

Gandhi S, Felini MJ, Nidetan H, Cardarelli K, Jadhav S, Faramawi M, Johnson ES (2014) A pilot case cohort study of brain cancer in poultry and control workers. Nutr Cancer. https://www.ncbi.nlm.nih.gov/pubmed/24564367

Professor Johnson, an epidemiologist at the University of Fort Worth Texas, has published more than 30 articles in scientific journals about increased cancer risks for employees in the meat industry, many of which are specifically for poultry farmers. To definitively link the cancer risk to occupational exposure, he has developed and patented the only test to date that can detect the presence of carcinogenic viruses in the genome of tumor cells of workers with these cancers.

Global differences in human diseases

Increased consumption of energy, animal proteins, animal fats and red meat was produced in different regions of the world after the transition to a more industrialized diet, hamburgers, sugary drinks and fast food in these countries.

USA
Western Europe
The Netherlands
Middle East
India
China
East Asia, Japan and Korea
Polynesia

USA

With more than 225 million overweight people in 2016, the USA has the largest number of overweight people in the world. The USA also export these unhealthy eating habits around the world. Worse diet is the leading cause of morbidity and mortality in the United States. With an average life expectancy of 78.1 years the United States comes in only at number fifty of the world ranking list, despite being the richest nation on the planet with the most advanced medical technology. The Netherlands is slightly better with an average life expectancy of 79.2 years, less than most other European countries. Even in spite of the nation's alarming high suicide rate Japanese live 82.1 years on average.

Diseases relating to diet are the leading causes of death to the United States. The number of people overweight or obese increased between 1990 and 2016. In the most comprehensive study of US health to date, poor diet was found to be the leading cause of morbidity and mortality, even surpassing smoking. Poor diet contributed to 14 percent, while smoking accounted for 11 percent. Obesity and high blood pressure accounted for 11 and eight percent respectively. The number one cause of death in America is the American diet. High blood pressure by fifty-five, heart attacks at sixty, maybe even cancer at seventy, and so on... For most of the leading causes of death, the science shows that the genes often account for only 10-20% of the risk at most. For example, when people move from low risk to high risk countries, their disease rates almost always change to those of the new environment. New diet, new diseases. But the reverse is also true. If we're eating the Standard American Diet and switch to a diet higher in whole plant foods, such as fruits and vegetables, this may lower your risk.

Western Europe

Europeans could spread at the expense of other peoples by infecting them (usually unintentionally) with epidemic infectious diseases such as smallpox and measles, to which Europeans had developed some genetic resistance and had acquired a lot of (anti-antibody) resistance. The exchange of major epidemic infectious diseases was one-sided, as most of those diseases came from the temperate zones of livestock farming (such as cattle, pigs and chickens) with which our forefathers lived in close contact after domestication of those animals. Of the 14 species of mammals valuable for animal husbandry in the world, 13 were Eurasian, only one American and none Australian. That is why Eurasians have developed resistance to their own diseases as disease carriers.

(Guns, Germs and Steel: The Fates of Human Society. Jared Diamond 1997.

Cancer is now the most common cause of death in Western Europe, more often than chronic obstructive pulmonary disease (COPD) and cardiovascular disease and diabetes (IHD). While mortality rates for COPD and IHD are declining due to improved health care, mortality rates for cancer have increased. Our Western eating habits and addiction to animal proteins in the form of ground beef, hamburgers and all kinds of meat products are the cause of the increase in cancer. The production of meat (products), poultry, pork and other meat tripled between 1980 and 2010 and is likely to double again by 2050. In 2050 there will be 500 million more cattle, 200 million more pigs, 1 billion more sheep and goats and 18 billion extra poultry than in 2005.

The Netherlands

Country	Cigarette packs of 20 per year in 1970	Lung cancer mortality 1984 (CBS NL)	2010 (EUROSTAT)
Italy	84	77	73
Norway	88	43	71
France	92	65	87
Finland	93	87	73
Netherlands	**108**	**117**	**108**
Belgium	**119**	**119**	**115**
West Germany	125	73	West & East Germany 79
Japan	*141*	*43*	
United Kingdom	**153**	**100**	**82**
USA	*184*	*84*	

Age standardized lung cancer mortality (ICD 162 per 100,000 men per year) in ten different countries in 1984, 2007 and 2010 in relation to per adult consumption of manufactured / hand-rolled cigarettes in 1970.

- **In Japan and the USA (see the table) has always been a lot more smoking and mortality rates of lung cancer were much lower.**

In 2012, cancer was the cause of 31% of all deaths in the Netherlands (Eurostat). Today about half of all men and one third of all women develop cancer and about 20% of all deaths are due to cancer. This is an impressive increase and seems to show that the increase in cancer is a recent biological event.

- Most lung cancer in the Netherlands, Belgium and the
  United Kingdom. These three countries have the largest share
  in the international trade and import of tropical birds via
  Amsterdam Schiphol, Brussels Zaventhem and London
  Heathrow respectively.

Bird exhibitions and bird breeders caused an explosive growth

Since the slave trade and slavery were abolished 150 years ago, international trade in tropical companion animals, international human trafficking, the arms industry and drug trafficking became the most profitable forms of trade. Worldwide, an estimated 40,000 primates, 4 million exotic birds, 640,000 reptiles and 350 million tropical fish are traded live each year. The trade in exotics is estimated at an $ 6 billion industry. Bird exhibitions and bird breeders caused an explosive growth of this popular hobby

Keeping and breeding tropical birds is a hobby of young families. The ratio of breeders to the total number of bird keepers is about 1: 6. The level of organization of the large bird breeders in the Netherlands is high due to participation in the breeding competitions. Public shows, which were held several times a year, made the hobby increasingly popular in the twentieth century. When pigeons are kept together with tropical birds, Chlamydia infections are more common.

In the Netherlands were 7.5 million birds in households in 1984. The American Veterinary Medicine Association (AVMA) counted 11-16 million companion birds and exotic birds in the United States in 2007. In France, 6 million companion birds were owned by households in 2010. In Belgium every bred bird must be provided with a ring with a number to which the owner can identify the breeder. In 2011 the Association Ornithologique de Belgique (AOB) registered 249 ornithological associations, authorized to identify their birds by an official ring. Pet birds are a lucrative business for pet stores and local breeders, as a single male canary is already sold for around 30 euros in

Belgium and a female for about 20 euros. Prices are about the same for zebra finches and budgerigars, and 50% to 100% higher for "special" finches such as bullfinches. Bird fairs and markets for live birds also attract many people. In addition, some species are bred because of their very high value; for example, in the case of canaries, the male and female specimens with particular genetic potential are presented in the national and international competitions for their posture (the Bossu Belge), the color (red mosaic) or for their song (Harzer). Consequently, the offspring can be sold for strongly increased prices. Baby parrots are quickly removed from the nest and, for example, with syringes fed by hobby breeders. A parrot reacts like a peewit: when eggs are taken away, she puts extra for. Growers get that way not three but six eggs per round. That saves quite a lot of money. The African Grey parrot quickly produces 700 euros. The doll, the female parrot, is literally milked and is not growing old.

Several times a year these beautiful birds are brought to shows and competitions, to exchange or sell. Exotic birds such as larger parrots, macaw or cockatoo are traded legally or illegally from Asia or South America. These birds are still high on the list of popular pets and are also richly represented in zoos and parks.

Tropical birds and pigeons transmit diseases to humans

From the infectious diseases transmitted by cage birds to humans, a number have been adapted so that they can pass from human to human and cause epidemics. This also infects people who do not keep or breed birds.

- Highly contagious Parrot Disease (Chlamydia psittaci), Ornithosis (Chlamydia pneumoniae) and Pneumonia (Chlamydia pneumoniae and TWAR)
- Infectious inflammatory bowel disease caused by Salmonella typhimurium
- Contagious bird flu (Influenza A(viair) Virus H5N1 - H7N9)

Chlamydia pneumoniae is nowadays an important cause of pneumonia. Chronic infection with Cp can cause lung cancer, cardiovascular disease and Alzheimer's disease. Chlamydia pneumoniae (Cp) infections initially had a mild course. With recurrence, more serious symptoms occur. This small, sneaky bacterium causes acute respiratory diseases and up to 20% of pneumonia in adults. The domestic form developed the ability to easily spread from person to person. Almost everyone can expect to be infected with Cp at least once during their lifetime and infections can become chronic. Recontamination during the term is common, especially among bird keepers and bird breeders. Chlamydia psittacosis has adapted in Western Europe and ornithosis and Chlamydia pneumonia were the result of this. Chlamydia pneumoniae is the humanized form of the zoonotic Chlamydia psittaci -> ornithosis -> TWAR -> Chlamydia pneumoniae. Chlamydia psittaci has managed to adapt and is today a communicable disease from person to person via the respiratory tract and has spread widely in society (Grayston JT). The original source has been the import of large numbers of tropical birds from South America and the breeding of tropical birds often in combination with a carrier pigeon hobby.

Pigeons sport

The Dutch Post Pigeon Organization (NPO) in Utrecht had 55,000 members in 1982, with an average of 30 carrier pigeons (100 after the breeding season). The members of the NPO have about 1 - 2 million pigeons with each other, depending on the season. Members act among themselves and with the fans of the sport in Belgium. There are almost no commercial racing pigeon dealers, unless a bird trader happens to be breeding pigeons himself. The breeding of racing pigeons has become an addiction among enthusiasts. The real pigeon keeper knows each of his birds and spends most of his free time in the loft. He places bets on the performance of his birds and can reclaim his investment many times when his bird finishes first. There is a well-developed system of leg rings and time clocks.

Especially, when racing pigeons or fancy pigeons are kept with other birds, they spread all kinds of bird flu. When transporting for trade, or during day trips, which make pigeons many times a year to Belgium, France, Spain or England, the birds are sent in large baskets, where there is ample opportunity for a wide spread of contaminated excrement. Previously it was thought that imported, often illegal birds, were the main source for distribution, but many domestic birds and pigeons bred in their own country have now also become infected. In 2010, the presence of the parrot disease bacteria was investigated in 32 Belgian pigeon breeding stocks and 61 wild-flying pigeons that were caught in the city of Ghent, Belgium. In addition, the transfer of the bacteria was examined in these breeding files. Carriers were often infected, at least one of the lofts was positive in 13 of the 32 (40.6%) pigeon loft stocks. Human infection was discovered in 4 of the 32

(12.5%) pigeon fanciers. This study clearly shows the possible risk of transmission of pigeons to humans from the tropical parrot bacterium.

- Pigeon breeders often use (37.5%) antibiotics for the prevention of respiratory diseases.

In a patient-controlled study in Scottish hospitals (Gardiner AJ 1992) 143 lung cancer patients of all ages were compared with 143 controls with cardiovascular disease and 143 controls with orthopedic disorders. They found a 3.9 times increased risk of lung cancer in keeping pigeons; for the younger age group 55-64 years they found a significantly increased risk of lung cancer in connection with keeping pigeons 5.62 times more (95% CI 1.58-20). Probably there were more active pigeon breeders in the younger age group.

Indoor air pollution

Significantly increased dust levels are measured in households where birds are kept. Particulate matter with a diameter of 2.5 micron or less is the most important health risk of (indoor) air pollution. The number of particles of about 2 microns is increased in bird-keeping households. Bird keepers, and especially bird breeders, have an increased risk of infection with local damage to the tissue and allergic reactions in the lung tissue. Due to excessive mucus production, there is more drainage of alveoli in smokers than in non-smokers. As a result, the dust container and antigen load is shifted from the alveoli to the smaller air tubes in the bird keeper who smokes. The antigens reach the smallest alveoli in smaller quantities and the immune responses and inflammation occur more strongly in smaller bronchi.

- **The smaller bronchi are the preferred location of lung cancer**

Both smoking and keeping birds are ultimately responsible for the poor functioning of the "lung cleaning service" and a shortage of immune proteins. The result is less protection of the lung mucosal cells against continual allergen and fine material that precipitates on the thin mucus layer of the smaller air tubes and subsequently lung cancer. It is therefore possible to see why most lung tumors develop in the smaller air tubes, at some distance from the finest alveoli, where gases and dust particles circulate at first instance. Both smoking and keeping birds at home increases the dust content of the air in the house.

- **Dust particles from bird cages and tobacco smoke are potentially more harmful than the particles that occur in outside air (eg pollen grains, ash, soot particles and sand grains)**

- There is every reason to pay particular attention to the bird breeders among the smokers.

Felderhof-Hoytema (1987) followed 699 school children aged 4 to 16 in The Hague. Of these children, 39.6% had birds at home. In children with one or more cage birds at home, 50.9% had symptoms of Chronic Non-Specific Lung Disease compared to 19% in children without cage birds at home. Converted, this means that 50% of the more serious forms of CNSLD, are related to the presence of cage birds at home.

- It is more obvious to measure particulate matter levels in households with birds than in classrooms.

Lung Cancer in the Netherlands

As a general practitioner I asked myself in the 1970s, why is it that so many people get prematurely ill and die before the age of 60? The search began for me after the first ten lung cancer patients I encountered. Of these, 6 were bird keepers / breeders.

Higher mortality before the age of 60 among those who kept and bred birds

During the survey period 28 deaths occurred before age 60 years, of which 19 were in men and 9 in women. There was no significant increase in death rates among those who kept dogs, cats or rodents, but there was a significant increase, in males and in both sexes, among those who kept birds. There were ten deaths in patients who had intensive contact with birds. Three cases stand out:

- The boy, who died at the age of 17 from a bone cancer in his leg, kept and bred continuously at least 100 tropical songbirds in a basement. You can imagine his risk of repeated bird flu and the occurrence of blood and bone marrow sepsis with slow persistent infection.
- One couple was examined from 1971 to 1979 after 3 years of marriage. The man had oligospermia. In 1976 the man had an aspecific lung infiltrate and from this time onwards epileptic seizures. In 1984 the man died aged 47 years from an ethmoid sinus carcinoma. No children were born (gravida 0). Before marriage the man had an aviary with a parrot and budgerigars and a dovecote. After marriage, the couple kept and bred about 15 pairs of canaries on their top floor permanently.
- Another couple was examined from 1975 to 1980 after 6 years of marriage. The man had ejaculatory impotence. In April 1980 the man, aged 32, sudden died while jogging in

the dunes. Post-mortem examination showed aortic valve stenosis with calcification and signs of endocarditis. No children were born. The man kept and bred birds in his youth and had an aviary in his bedroom over his folding bed with many pairs of tropical birds. His father died from lung cancer at the age of 50 years. After the couple married, they kept a parrot, a Japanese nightingale, two budgerigars and a Mozambique.

Lung Cancer risk for men under 65 years of age was increased six-fold in those who kept birds

Both in the hospital case-control study and in the general practice survey in the Hague, lung cancer risk for men under 65 years of age was increased six-fold in those who had kept birds as pets 5 – 14 years before diagnosis of the lung cancer. This finding, coupled with the fact that one household in three or four keeps birds, implies that more than 50% of the total lung cancer rate in men under 65 years of age in The Hague can be attributed to keeping/breeding birds.

The finding of a relation between lung cancer and bird keeping/ breeding for men under 65 years of age is supported by a study in West Berlin (Kohlmeier L 1992). Two studies found a relation for lung cancer patients below 55 years of age (Jöckel KH 2002, Kocazeybek B 2003). The study in Scotland (Gardiner AJ 1992) found a significant relation with pigeon keeping for patients 55-64 years of age. And the study in Taipei (Ger LP 1992) found also a significant relation between pigeon keeping and lung cancer. Anttila TI 2003, in a prospective study of Finnish women, found also a significant relation between Chlamydia pneumoniae infection and lung cancer, also among the nonsmoking women.

Experimental induction of lung cancer

Chronic inhalation studies with cigarette smoke machines, in hamsters, dogs and monkeys showed no statistically significant increase in malignant tumors in the airways, although very long exposures and high doses of smoke were used (Coggins CR 2001). These inhalation studies were performed without concomitant infection of the airways of the laboratory animals. The tobacco industry has long cited the studies as evidence for no increase in lung cancer due to smoking.

Recently (Chu DJ 2012) a lung cancer animal model was developed through repeated injection of Chlamydia pneumonia in airways of rats, with or without benzo(a)pyrene. With the combination of benzo(a)pyrene and the bacteria of tropical bird flu in the spray, 44% of the laboratory rats got lung cancer.

- **Chlamydia pneumoniae of the bird cages have proven to be an independent risk factor for lung cancer**

The combined factors of smoking and Cp chronic infection have superimposed effects and lead to greatly increased lung cancer risk.

Chu DJ, Guo SG, Pan CF, Wang J, Du Y, Lu XF, Yu ZY (2012) An experimental model for induction of lung cancer in rats by Chlamydia pneumoniae. Asian Pac J Cancer Prev. 2012;13(6):2819-22
https://www.ncbi.nlm.nih.gov/pubmed/22938465

Follow-up references lung cancer studies

Anttila TI, Koskela P, Leinonen M et al. (2003) Chlamydia pneumoniae Infection and the Risk of Female Early-Onset Lung Cancer. Int J Cancer:107,681-682

https://www.ncbi.nlm.nih.gov/pubmed/14520711

Bruu AL, Haukenes G, Aasen S, Grayston JT, Wang SP, Klausen OG, Myrmel H, Hasseltvedt V (1991) Chlamydia pneumoniae infections in Norway 1981-87 earlier diagnosed as ornithosis. Scand J Infect Dis 23(3):299-304

Chaturvedi AK et al. (2010) Chlamydia pneumoniae infection and risk for lung cancer. Cancer Epidemiol Biomarkers Prev 1498-1505

https://www.ncbi.nlm.nih.gov/pubmed/20501758

Chu DJ, Guo SG, Pan CF, Wang J, Du Y, Lu XF, Yu ZY (2012) An experimental model for induction of lung cancer in rats by Chlamydia pneumoniae. Asian Pac J Cancer Prev. 2012;13(6):2819-22

https://www.ncbi.nlm.nih.gov/pubmed/22938465

Chu DJ, Yao DE, Zhuang YF, Hong Y, Zhu XC, Fang ZR, Yu J and Yu ZY (2014) Azithromycin enhances the favorable results of paclitaxel and cisplatin in patients with advanced non-small cell lung cancer. Genet. Mol. Res. 13(2):2976-2805

https://www.ncbi.nlm.nih.gov/pubmed/24782093

Coggins CR (2001) A review of chronic inhalation studies with mainstream cigarette smoke, in hamsters, dogs, and nonhuman primates. Toxicol Pathol. 2001 Sep-Oct;29(5):550-7

Felini M, Preacely N, Shah N, Christopher A, Sarda V, Elfaramawi M, Sall M, Bangara S, Gandhi S, **Johnson ES** (2012) A case-cohort study of lung cancer in poultry and control workers: occupational findings. Occup Environ Med. 2012 Mar;69(3):191-7

Ferreri AJ, Dolcetti R, **Magnino** S ey al. (2007) A woman and her canary: a tale of chlamydiae and lymphomas. J Natl Cancer Inst. 2007 Sep 19;99(18):1418-9 https://www.ncbi.nlm.nih.gov/pubmed/17848672

Gardiner AJ, Forey AB, Lee PN (1992) Avian exposure and bronchiogenic carcinoma. Br Med J 305 :989-992

https://www.ncbi.nlm.nih.gov/pubmed/1458146

Ger LP, Liou SH, Shen CV, Kao SJ, Chen KT (1992) Risk factors of lung cancer.J. Formos Med Assoc Sep; 91 Suppl 3:222-231

https://www.ncbi.nlm.nih.gov/pubmed/1362909

Holst PAJ 1997 Risk of lung cancer needs to be studied in younger patients who keep and breed pet birds. Br Med J (1997) 314, 1353

Jackson LA, Wang SF, Nazar-Stewart V, Grayston IT, Vaughan IL (2000) Association of Chlamydia pneumoniae immunoglobin A seropositivity and risk of lung cancer. Cancer Epidemiol Biomarkers Prev 9(11): 1263-1266
https://www.ncbi.nlm.nih.gov/pubmed/11097237

Johnson ES, Ndetan H, Lo KM (2010) Cancer mortality in poultry slaughtering / processing plant workers belonging a union pension fund. Environ Res 110(6):588-94
https://www.ncbi.nlm.nih.gov/pubmed/20541185

Johnson ES (2012), Choi Km. Lung cancer risk in workers in the meat and poultry industries - a review. Zoonoses Public Health 59(5):303-13
https://www.ncbi.nlm.nih.gov/pubmed/22332987

Jöckel KH, Pohlabeln H, Bromen K, Ahrens W, Jahn I (2002) Pet Birds and risk of lung cancer in North-Western Germany. Lung Cancer Jul;37(1)29-34

Kocazeybek B (2003) Chronic Chlamydophila pneumoniae infection in lung cancer, a risk factor: a case-control study. J Med Microbiol 52(8):721-6

Kohlmeier L, Arminger A, Bartolomeycik S, Bellach B, Rehm J, Thamm M (1992) Pet birds as an independent risk for lung cancer: Case-control study. Br Med J 305:986-989 https://www.ncbi.nlm.nih.gov/pubmed/1458145

Koyi H, Branden E, Gnarpe J, Gnarpe H, Arnholm B, Hillerdal G (1999) Chlamydia pneumoniae may be associated with lung cancer. Preliminary report on a seroepidemiological study. APMlS 107(9):828

Laurilla AL, Antilla T, Laara E, Bloigu A, Virtamo J, Albanes D, Leinonen M, Saikku P (1997) Serological evidence of an association between Chlamydia pneumoniae infection and lung cancer. Int J Cancer 20;74(1)1-34

Littman AJ Jackson LA, Vaughan TL (2005) Chlamydia pneumoniae and lung cancer: epidemiologic evidence. Cancer Epidemiol Biomarkers Prev. 14(4):773-8
https://www.ncbi.nlm.nih.gov/pubmed/15824142

Mather JP, Roberts PE, Pan Z et al. (2013) Isolation of cancer stem like cells from human adenosquamous carcinoma of the lung supports a monoclonal origin from a multipotential tissue stem cell. PLoS One 4;8(12)

Zhan P, Suo LJ, Qian Q, Shen XK, Qiu LX, Yu LK, Song Y (2011). Chlamydia pneumoniae infection and lung cancer risk: a meta-analysis. Eur J Cancer Mar;47(5):742-7
https://www.ncbi.nlm.nih.gov/pubmed/21194924

Middle East

In 2013, when I flew over the Arabian Peninsula, I saw the integrated crop circles of Saudi Arabia. Saudi farmers feed the production of grains in the desert by winning underground water supplies. Part of that water dates back 20,000 years, until the last ice age, when more moderate conditions filled aquifers. On the ground these circles are as wide as the water-bearing layers deep, about one kilometer. Sprinklers with central pivotal pits draw from the groundwater. Many of the crops are grown to feed the intensive livestock industry. Camels are rarely used as a means of transport. Dromedary camels are bred for their milk and meat and to participate in camel races. The Saudi kingdom has implemented a multi-faceted program to supply large quantities of water, necessary to realize the spectacular growth of the agricultural sector. Vast underground water reservoirs have been drained through deep wells, the desert was transformed into fertile farmland.

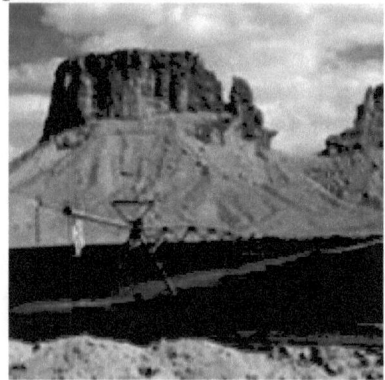

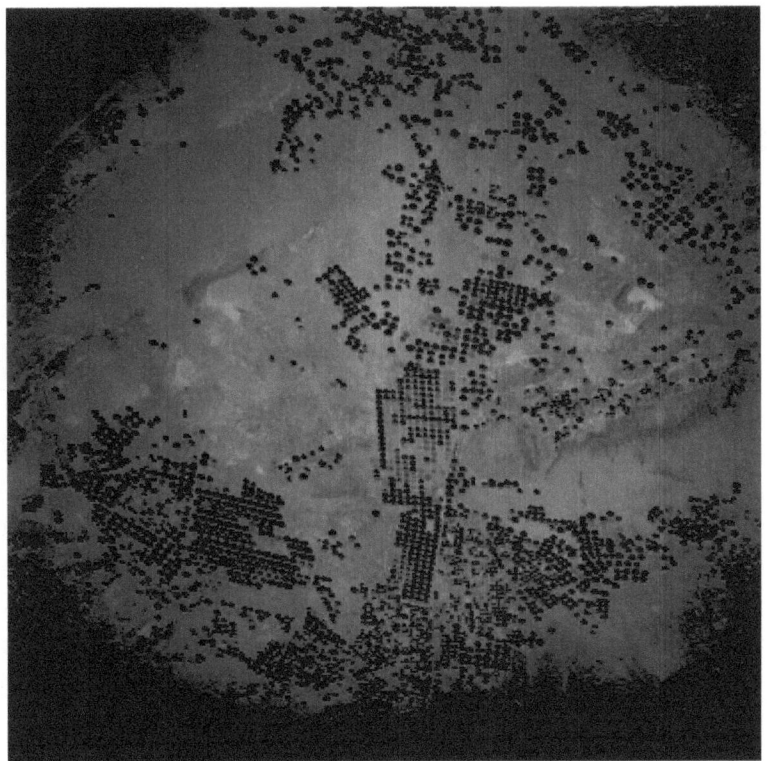

Crop circles on the Arab peninsula

Dromedary flu, from virus-spreading young camels, is the result of intensive camel breeding on the Arab peninsula. There is a rapid increase in the number of reported infections with Middle East Respiratory Syndrome Corona Virus (MERS-CoV). Since June 2012, MERS-CoV has infected more than 1,814 people, with 734 deaths (41%). The disease first occurred on the Arabian Peninsula, in Saudi Arabia and the United Arab Emirates. Concerns about the situation have increased considerably, particularly concerns about the spread of the infection in hospitals and in contacts with patients. Dromedary camel flu is endemic among young dromedary camels in Saudi Arabia. Sick camels separate corona viruses from their noses and sometimes in feces. Only recently people and dromedary camels share the same corona viruses. The corona virus first adapted in the herds of camel breeders, with larger concentrations of young dromedary camels. The breeding and weaning season is a factor. Young camels are more susceptible to camel flu because of their lower immunity status and they promote virus amplification. Today the MERS-CoV circulates from person to person and is less virulent. These humanized corona viruses pass through the airways and are increasingly common in society. Without stopping the transmission of these camel flu, we will continue to see more human cases in the Middle East. With the annual Hajj Pilgrimage to Mecca in October, more than 2 million Muslims from more than 180 countries are at risk of receiving MERS-CoV and spreading it to their home countries. Saudi authorities warn their citizens against drinking unpasteurized camel milk and advise them to wear gloves when they care for the animals. The omnipresence of the animals, their importance for the economy of the region and their popularity mean that the transfer of MERS-CoV to the camels to humans will continue to take place. The father of the current Syrian president promised his people full granaries and more meat pots. In Syria too, water sources were tapped to promote agriculture and livestock farming. A drought period and shortages of water drove the farming population en masse to the cities. Great social unrest ensued. The popular uprising in Syria is brutally precipitated. Poverty, war, hunger, higher temperatures, drought and lack of water mean that more and more people are fleeing from the Middle East and Central Africa.

India

U.S. men get 23 times more prostate cancer than men in India. Americans get between 8 and 14 times the rate of melanoma, 10 to 11 times more colorectal cancer, 9 times more endometrial cancer, 7 to 17 times more lung cancer, 7 to 8 times more bladder cancer, 5 times more breast cancer, and 9 to 12 times more kidney cancer. This is not mere 5, 10, or 20 percent more, but 5, 10, or 20 times more. Hundreds of percent more breast cancer, thousands of percent more prostate cancer, differences greater than those found in the China Study.

Because Indians account for one-sixth of the world's population, and have some of the highest spice consumption in the world, epidemiological studies in this country have great potential for improving our understanding of the relationship between diet and cancer. The lower rates of cancer may, of course, not be due to higher spice intake. Several dietary factors may contribute to the low overall rate of cancer in India. Among them are a "relatively low intake of meat and a mostly plant-based diet, in addition to the high intake of spices." Forty percent of Indians are vegetarian, and even the ones that do eat meat don't eat a lot. And it's not only what they don't eat, but what they do. India is one of the largest producers and consumers of fresh fruits and vegetables, and Indians eat a lot of pulses (legumes), such as beans, chickpeas, and lentils. They also eat a wide variety of spices in addition to curcuma that constitute, by weight, the most anti-oxidant-packed class of foods in the world (Holt PR).

China

It is very unfortunate that the Year of the Rat 2020 in China starts with a new coronavirus epidemic, caused by bats, also known as the flying rats. Chinese eat everything that has legs attached to it, except chairs. People in many parts of the world eat bats, and sell them in live animal markets, which was the source of SARS and the latest coronavirus epidemic that began in Wuhan. At the Wuhan live market exotic animals as snakes, turtles, bats, foxes and porcupines are sold for consumption. Even civets, a cat-like creature, were still among dozens of species listed on an exhaustive price list for one of the animal trading businesses at the Wuhan market. Bats are host to a higher proportion of zoonoses than all other mammals. They are also an incredible diverse group, making up about a quarter of all mammalian species. Their ability to coexist with viruses that can spill over to other mammals, in particular humans, can have devastating consequences when we eat them, trade them in livestock markets, and invade their territory.

- Stopping the sale of wildlife in markets is essential to curtail future outbreaks of diseases that spill over from animals to humans.
- **The decision, taken by the Chinese National People's Congress on February 24, 2020, that illegal consumption and trade in wild animals will be "severely punished", as well as hunting, trade or transportation of wild animals for consumption is a good start.**

Far East, Japan and Korea

In Japan and Korea, large-scale imports of beef and pork began after the Second World War, respectively after the Korean War. In 1970 in Japan and 1990 in Korea a sharp increase in the numbers of colon cancer was observed. Consumption of fried beef (eg shabu-shabu, Korean yukhoe and Japanese yukke) became very popular in both countries. A specific meat factor, presumably one or more thermo-resistant potential carcinogenic bovine viruses (for example polyoma, papilloma or single-stranded DNA viruses), can contaminate the beef and lead to latent infections in the intestinal tract.

zur Hausen H (2012) Red meat consumption and cancer: reasons for suspect involvement or bovine infectious factors in colorectal cancer. Int J Cancer. 2012 Jun 1; 130 (11): 2475-83

https://www.ncbi.nlm.nih.gov/pubmed/22212999

Increased consumption of energy, animal fat and red meat has occurred in East Asia in recent decades. Data on breast cancer, colon, prostate, esophagus and stomach cancer mortality rates for China (1988-2000), Hong Kong (1960-2006), Japan (1950-2006), Korea (1985-2006) and Singapore (1963- 2006) were obtained from the WHO. In the selected countries (except breast cancer in Hong Kong), a noticeable increase in mortality rates of breast, colon and prostate cancer and a decreasing decrease in esophageal and gastric cancer in the study periods were observed. For example, the annual percentage increase in mortality in breast cancer was 5.5% for the period 1985-1993 in Korea and the mortality rates for prostate cancer increased from 1958 to 1993 in Japan by 3.2% per year. These changes in cancer mortality followed ~ 10 years after the transition to more industrially prepared food, hamburgers, sugary drinks and fast food in these countries.

Zhang J, Dhakai IB, Zhao Z, Li L (2012) Trends in mortality from cancers of the breast, colon, prostate, esophagus, and stomach in East Asia: role of nutrition transition. Eur J Cancer Prev 2012 Sep; 21 (5): 480-9

https://www.ncbi.nlm.nih.gov/pubmed/22357483

Mortality rates for prostate cancer have increased dramatically (25x) in Japan after the Second World War. After the war the consumption of milk increased by 20x, from meat 9x and from eggs 7x. Milk contains large amounts of estrogens plus proteins and saturated fats. The recent increase in its use is likely to be the cause of the surge of prostate cancer in Japan.

Ganmaa D, Li XM, Qin LQ et al. The experience of Japan as a clue to the etiology of testicular and prostatic cancers. Med Hypotheses. 2003 May; 60 (5): 724-30

https://www.ncbi.nlm.nih.gov/pubmed/12710911

Japan is the country with the most centenarians in the world in 2016. The story of these centenarians and their daily habits are different of the western way of life.

Polynesia

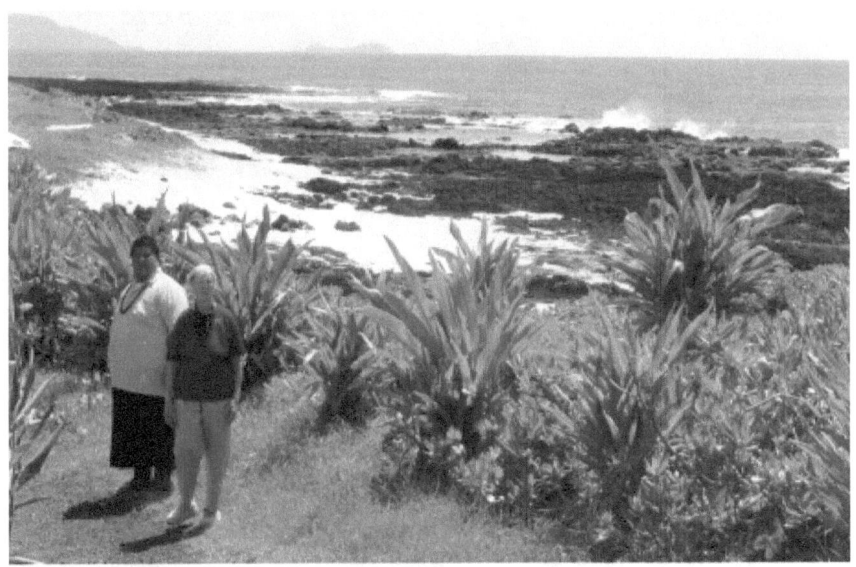

The inhabitants of Tuvalu, Fiji, Samoa and the Cook Islands are massively overweight. According to the World Health Organization (WHO), nine of the world's ten thickest countries belong to the Pacific Islands. Tonga (4th, 90.8%), Samoa (6th, 80.4%) and USA (9th, 74.1%). Up to 95 percent of the adult population is overweight in some countries. The number of people with obesity, extremely overweight, varies from 35 to 50 percent. The Cook Islands (90.9% overweight) are in third place in the world ranking. Slightly more than half of the population suffers from obesity. There are several reasons for this. First, being fat is more accepted. In Polynesia the perception of "big is beautiful" actually prevails. Inexpensive factory processed food has replaced the original diet of fresh fish and vegetables. Fresh fish is relatively expensive, with this money you can buy multiple hamburger meals. A bottle of cola is cheaper here than a bottle of water. 75% of the women on Samoa are extremely overweight.

https://youtu.be/RSwpX15ZNcA

Smoking addiction

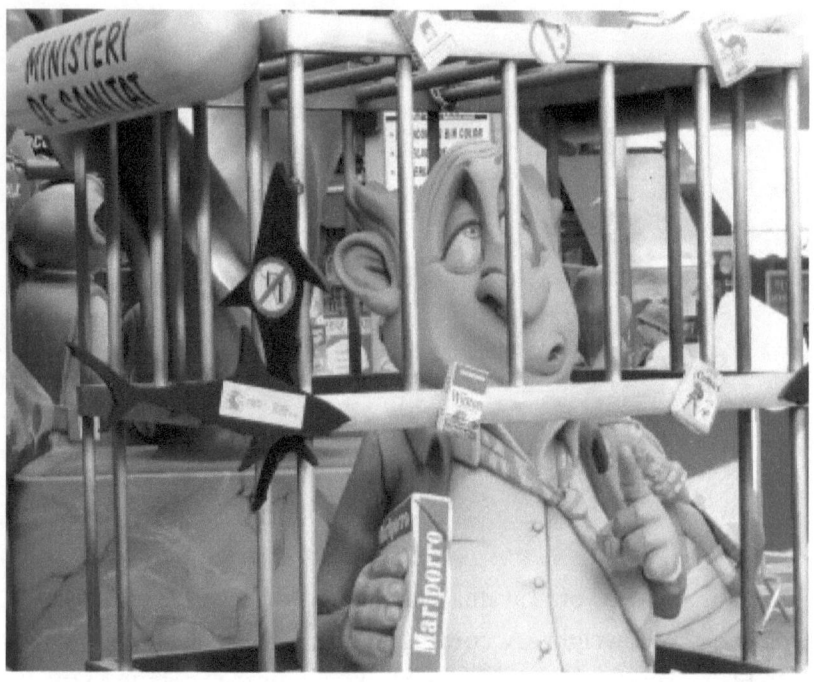

- We are all exposed to cigarette smoke and, in particular, to one of the most important carcinogenic ingredients: benzo (a) pyrene.
- Smokers who breathe deep into the smoke and hold the smoke in their lungs for 2 - 3 seconds, by breathing out slowly, have a larger deposit of particles of 1 - 3 μm in their airways. The process of absorption of water vapor by hygroscopic particles in cigarette smoke is recognizable.

- A smoker who breathes long and deep, blows out white smoke instead of the blue smoke that is the original color of tobacco burning gases

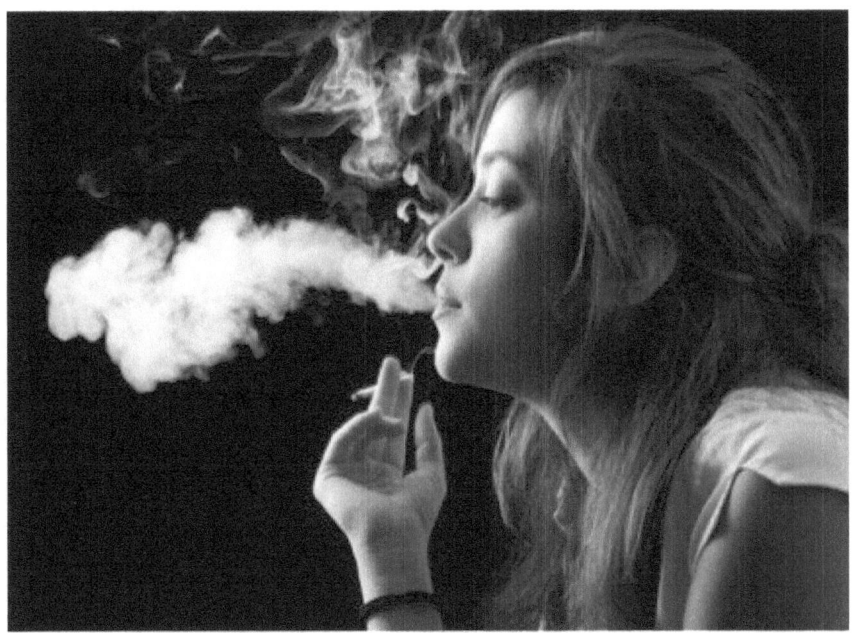

Irritation of the respiratory tract mucous membrane as a result of smoking leads to increased mucous production. In the long run, the heavy smoker's first cigarette of the morning does not produce enough irritation to cough up all the mucus that has collected during the night. A drainage problem arises on the minute air sacs involving stasis and a diminution of the diameter of the smaller bronchi. Stasis increases the risk of infection and allergic processes if inhaled micro-organisms and antigens can reach these areas. Some smokers cough and bring up mucus. Some develop a severe bronchial obstructive syndrome, in which coughing is completed with shortness of breath and wheezing in the chest. In addition to accumulation of mucus, these patients have bronchial spasms and edema of the bronchial mucous membrane and muscles of the bronchial wall, and to allergic processes in the bronchial wall.

- **Smokers with shortness of breath, coughs and wheezing in the chest are individuals who develop the most lung** tumors

Bio-industry

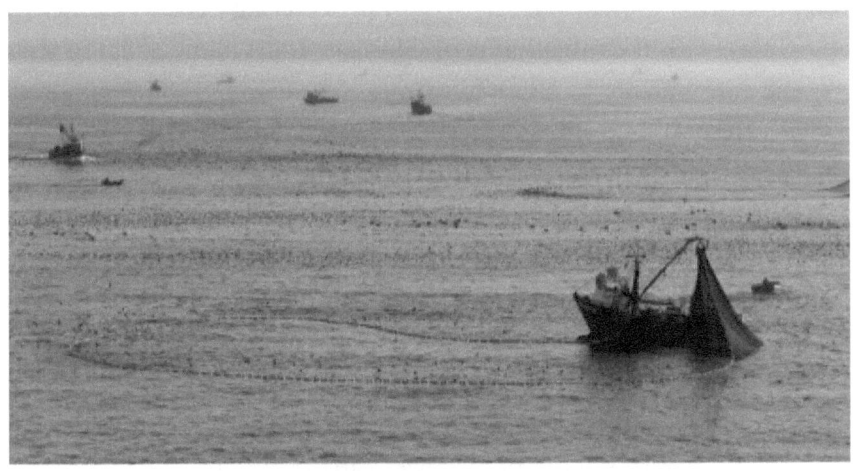

Anchovy from the southeast of the Pacific Ocean is sold as cattle feed to Europe's factory farms. Approximately one third of the total catch is fed to consumption animals, mostly farmed fish, pigs and chickens. European fishermen are obliged to land all by-catches by 2020. In addition to the by-catches, the fish-processing industry also produces a significant amount of reusable waste, such as skins, bones, fish heads and internal organs. Fish meal can be created by hydrolysis of the fish from the by-catches and fish remains, which is a great need. Especially at the fish farms in the Mediterranean. Tuna, salmon, cattle, pigs and chickens grow faster and fatter by fishmeal. More profit can be achieved and the time to slaughter is shortened. For production of fish oil and fishmeal, some 20-30 million tons of fish, anchovies, herring, mackerel and sprat species have been removed from the southeastern Pacific Ocean over the past decades. Consumption on a large scale of small glass eels, and of caviar, fish eggs, is also harmful to fish stocks.

Going back 1000 years in Europe, it was declines in freshwater fish thanks to human pressure which first pushed fishermen out into the oceans in larger numbers. Five hundred years ago, it was the decline of coastal fish that brought deep-sea trawling into existence. A hundred and fifty years ago there was still enough room on the planet. The population growth was still within the carrying capacity of the planet. Today, with the inhabitants of China or India alone equal to those of the entire planet in 1850, humanity has expanded to the point where we are crashing. The earth is overpopulated. As with agriculture, it is not the small businesses that consume the most aid, they are the industrial producers. Worldwide 20 billion is awarded annually. 6.3 billion is spent on subsidies for fuel alone; an extra 8 billion goes to the maintenance of the major ports. Small fishing uses 75% less energy to catch the same volume of fish, more environmentally friendly and with many more people. Abolish these subsidies and industrial fishing suddenly becomes a much less profitable business.

Mega farms with only cows, calves, pigs or chickens feed the animals with soy flour, fish meal and low doses of antibiotics to fatten the animals faster and to gain more profit. This has drastically increased the animal fat content of steak, pork and chicken meat. Welfare diseases such as cardiovascular diseases, increased blood pressure, excess weight and diabetes increase due to food with a high content of saturated animal fat.

Bowel Cancer

An increased risk of colorectal cancer has long been shown for the consumption of undercooked red meat. Fish and chicken do not increase this risk, although comparable or even higher concentrations of potentially cancer-causing chemicals are released during roasting or frying. In Japan and Korea, beef and pork were imported on a large scale after the Second World War and the Korean War. A strong increase in the number of patients with colon cancer was observed after 1970 in Japan and after 1990 in Korea. The consumption of undercooked beef (eg, Shabu-shabu, Korean Yukhoe and Japanese Yukke) became very popular in both countries.

Bovine leukemia virus as a source of colon cancer

A specific beef factor, probably one or more heat-resistant carcinogenic bovine viruses (for example, polyoma, papilloma or bovine leukemia virus BLV) can infect the beef and cause latent and persistent intestinal infections after human consumption (Zur Hausen H).

Polyoma viruses in hamburgers

In chopped beef samples three types of polyoma virus have been shown, which are resistant to BBQ temperatures and are carcinogenic to their natural hosts. Animal viruses are frequently found in meat products and can cause colon cancer in humans. The papilloma and polyoma viruses in particular are resistant to medium-heated steak tartar, in which the central parts of the meat are not heated above 40 - 70 degrees Celsius. These viruses endure 80 degrees Celsius for 30 minutes without losing too much of their ability to cause infections. These viruses are also insufficiently inactivated during the pasteurization of dairy products.

Acid-resistant bacteria and stomach cancer

Two Australian GPs realized that mycobacteria (acid-solid organisms) can survive the acidic environment of the stomach, which

83

other pathogenic bacteria cannot. They discovered one of the most important human pathogens, Helicobacter pylori, which are capable of causing severe stomach inflammatory disease. It was then discovered that these microbes cause gastric carcinoma.

Lichtman MA A Bacterial Cause of Cancer: An Historical Essay. Oncologist. 2017 May;22(5):542-548

https://www.ncbi.nlm.nih.gov/pubmed/28432224

Zhang J, Dhakai IB, Zhao Z, Li L (2012) Trends in mortality from cancers of the breast, colon, prostate, oesophagus, and stomach in East Asia: role of nutrition transition. Eur J Cancer Prev 2012 Sep;21(5):480-9

https://www.ncbi.nlm.nih.gov/pubmed/22357483

Zur Hausen H (2012) Red meat consumption and cancer: reasons to suspect involvement of bovine infectious factors in colorectal cancer. Int J Cancer.130(11):2475-83

https://www.ncbi.nlm.nih.gov/pubmed/22212999

Raw eggs and raw milk products

Insufficient heating of chicken egg proteins

Industrially processed food contains a large proportion of liquid chicken egg proteins that in some cases are not sufficiently heated processed. Eggs are released on crushers, egg yolk and white are separated, eggshells and hail cords are removed by filters and the protein product is heated to 56 ° Celsius. In the Netherlands (1983), 20,000 tons of liquid chicken protein was produced for the industry, which was marginally pasteurized sometimes insufficiently heat treated. The confectioner processes a large number of products that contain eggs. This can be the pasteurized proteins, or he processes fresh eggs. The "whites" are collected in a special container. Housewives also sometimes come into contact with raw egg proteins when making cake batter or desserts at home. Or if they whip up the raw egg proteins.

Raw egg proteins are processed in:

SUGAR GLAZE raw egg whites with powdered sugar

ROOM FONDANT raw egg whites with butter, sugar and liqueur

OMELET SIBÉRIEN raw egg whites with sugar

BAVAROIS raw egg whites with sugar, cream, gelatin, fruits

ICE CREAM raw egg whites with sugar, milk and cream.

And in:

STEAK TARTAR with a raw egg

Raw milk products

Raw milk is milk from cows, sheep, or goats that has not been pasteurized to kill harmful bacteria. This raw, unpasteurized milk can carry dangerous bacteria such as Salmonella, E. coli and Listeria, which are responsible for causing numerous foodborne illnesses. These harmful bacteria can seriously affect the health of anyone who drinks raw milk, or eats foods made from raw milk. However, the bacteria in raw milk can be especially dangerous to people with weakened immune systems, older adults, pregnant women, and children.

Pasteurization is a process that kills harmful bacteria by heating milk to a specific temperature for a set period of time; 1st developed by Louis Pasteur in 1864, pasteurization kills harmful organisms responsible for such diseases as listeriosis, typhoid fever, tuberculosis, diphtheria, and brucellosis. While pasteurization has helped provide safe, nutrient-rich milk and cheese for over 120 years, some people continue to believe that pasteurization harms milk and that raw milk is a safe, healthier alternative.

Myths and proven facts about milk and pasteurization:

- Pasteurizing milk DOES NOT cause lactose intolerance and allergic reactions. Both raw milk and pasteurized milk can cause allergic reactions in people sensitive to milk proteins.
- Raw milk DOES NOT kill dangerous pathogens by itself.
- Pasteurization DOES NOT reduce milk's nutritional value.
- Pasteurization DOES NOT mean that it is safe to leave milk out of the refrigerator for extended time, particularly after it has been opened.
- Pasteurization DOES kill harmful bacteria.
- Pasteurization DOES saves lives.

Breast Cancer

People are exposed to carcinogenic viruses that often occur in animals in the food chain, such as laying hens, eggs, broiler chickens and dairy cows. The Avian Leukemia Virus (ALV) and Bovine Leukemia Viruses (BLV) are RNA viruses and have been shown in breast cancer cells.

Bovine Leukemia Virus in breast cancer cells

Breast cancer and ovarian cancer were rare in Japan, compared with other countries. The mortality rates, however, are increasing. After the Second World War changes in lifestyle took place in Japan. In the past 50 years (1947-1997), mortality rates of breast and ovarian cancer increased 2- and 4-fold, and the respective intake of milk, meat and eggs increased 20, 10 and 7-fold. The increase in death rates from breast cancer and ovarian cancer could be attributed to the increased consumption of animal nutrition, which occurred after 1945. Milk, dairy products and eggs are probably the cause of this (Buehring). Cows are often infected with bovine leukemia virus (BLV), a carcinogenic virus that can be transferred from the cow to the calf via the milk or during birth. Most infected cattle seem healthy and the infection is persistent. Consumption of non-pasteurized dairy products, or cheese made from raw milk, or insufficiently heated beef at the BBQ can transmit this infectious virus to humans. About 38% of the cattle, 84% of the dairy herd, and 100% of factory farm herds in the US are infected with BLV. Less than 5% of these cattle get leukemia. With this condition the animals are not admitted to the US consumer market. The BLV virus circulates with the white blood cells through the blood of infected cattle. The BLV virus also infects the mammary gland cells of the cows and infected cells are found in cow's milk (Lanou AJ). Pasteurization of cow's milk makes the BLV ineffective.

Buehring GC (2015) has shown that 39% of people in a San Francisco Bay Area have antibodies against BLV in the blood, which is an indication of exposure to BLV. Almost all cow's milk contains BLV bovine leukemia virus. In a study of 213 women, BLV-related DNA was found in breast tissue of women with a diagnosis of breast cancer, not in breast tissue of women without history of breast cancer (Buehring).

Ovarian and fallopian tube cancer in laying hens

Ovarian cancer often occurs in laying hens (Frederickson TN). For this reason, they are usually slaughtered after the first leg year. In poultry farms, laying hens do not become older than 24 months. Avian Leukemia Virus (leucosis) is a retrovirus that infects large parts of the modern poultry farms and caused a lot of economic damage. The virus is present in chickens and eggs. Man is exposed to this. RNA viruses are single-stranded proteins that do not accurately divide. When RNA viruses divide within a host cell, they make many copies that differ from the original. Some of these copy differences increase their genetic variation and survival chances in the host. Therefore, although it is often possible to prevent a DNA virus infection with a sustainable vaccine, it is very difficult, if not impossible, to make a sustainable vaccine for an RNA virus, especially the RNA retroviruses. This also makes RNA viruses very difficult to treat with medicines.

Mice also infect the grain stocks with a virus that is closely related to breast cancer viruses (Stewart TH). Free-range chickens are often kept outside, so that the risk of contamination due to the contamination of food on the ground by mouse droppings is greater. In the winter months, mice often go to poultry farms to look for food. Virus spreading mice; contamination of cereals, chicken feeds and poultry; transfer by infected chickens from viruses to the eggs; processing of raw, insufficiently heated protein in confectionery products; this is how the ALV virus arrives in humans (Pham TD).

Raw proteins often contain leukemia virus (ALV and BLV)

Breast and colon cancer are not caused by breathing bad air. A causal relationship will be found earlier for pathogens in our diet. Animal proteins in milk and dairy products, in meat products and in egg proteins carry carcinogenic viruses. Improved laboratory techniques provide increasing evidence. A total of 22,788 persons with lactose intolerance were examined, who did not use milk products, and compared with people who did use milk products. The risk of lung, breast and colon cancer appeared to be significantly reduced in the group that did not use milk products. The risk of lung, breast and colon cancer appeared to be significantly reduced in the group that did not use milk products.

Ji J, Sundquist J, Sundquist K Lactose intolerance and reduced risk of lung, breast and ovarian cancers: aetiological clues from a population-based study in Sweden. Br J Cancer. 2015 Jan 6; 112 (1): 149-52

https://www.ncbi.nlm.nih.gov/pubmed/25314053

Breast cancer and ovarian cancer are they ZOONOSES?

The observation that chickens may be infected with a closely related form of mouse breast cancer virus (MMTV) may be of epidemiological significance for human breast cancer. Chickens and eggs can be infected by mice and in turn pass the virus on to people. The successful infection of human cells by MMTV has already been demonstrated (Indik S 2007). MMTV can infect human cell cultures and this finding provides a possible explanation for the discovery of MMTV in patients with breast cancer. The numbers of breast cancer that occur in humans vary geographically. No environmental factor could explain this variation. The highest incidence of breast cancer worldwide occurs in countries where Mus domesticus is the native or imported type of house mouse.

Stewart TH, Sage RD, Stewart AF, Cameron DW (2000) Breast cancer incidence highest in the range of one species of house mouse, Mus domesticus. Br J Cancer. 82(2):446-51.

https://www.ncbi.nlm.nih.gov/pubmed/10646903

Breast stem cells

Women who have remained childless have immature mammary cells with stem cell activity. When these cells become infected with carcinogenic virus, this infection leads to uncontrolled cell division. In the twentieth century, breast cancer was also called "the nuns disease." Full-term pregnancies reduce the risk of breast cancer and the higher the number of pregnancies, the greater this protection. The risk of breast cancer decreases by 7% after every full-term pregnancy. Women who have given birth to children have a 30% lower risk than childless women. Stem cells in the mammary gland are only developed after the first full-term pregnancy. Immature gland cells possess stem cell properties. The stem cell properties cause uncontrolled cell division at the time of infection or other forms of cell damage. The presence of breast cancer in the woman is closely related to her age. Breast cancer is most common in childless women and women around menopause. The biological regression of women begins around the time of menopause and is accompanied by a reduction of immune function of body cells. Reduced cell defenses can lead to the proliferation of infected mammary cells.

Melting glaciers

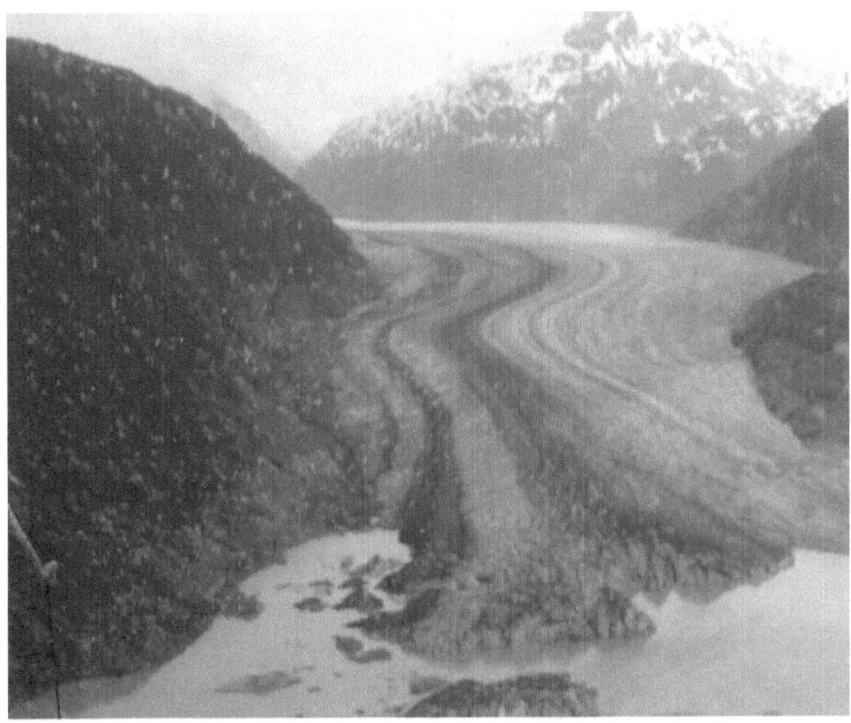

- Every year the glaciers in Alaska become hundreds of meters shorter by melting the ice. https://youtu.be/HY671_UR-qo
- In the USA, cattle emit approximately 5.5 million m3 of methane, a greenhouse 25 times more potent than CO2.

The fast-growing meat industry produces more greenhouse gases than the exhaust gases from all car traffic on earth. Melting glaciers are the result of this. Meat, milk and eggs in our food contribute more to the climate change in the world than the exhaust fumes of our fleet. Livestock farming accounts for at least 14.5% and, according to some studies, even 51% of man-made greenhouse gases. In the USA cattle emit approximately 5.5 million m3 of methane - a greenhouse gas that is 25 times more potent than CO2.

CE Delft, Fraunhofer Institute for Systems and Innovation Research and LEI Wageningen. Behavioural climate change mitigation options and their appropriate inclusion in quantitative longer-term policy scenarios. Delft, January 2012

All life depends on the oceans. Circulation in the North Atlantic has slowed to the lowest level in centuries. The slowdown of the Gulf Stream devastates fisheries and will lead to a rise in sea levels.

Large amounts of nitrogen from fertilizer and manure are distributed annually over agricultural land. No doubt that it increases crop yield, but plants do not absorb it completely, so that more fertilizer and animal waste is added than the plants need. Only a fraction of what is applied to the soil ends up in the crops. The rest flows to our rivers.

Nitrogen and phosphorus levels, dead organisms are increasing in the Gulf of Mexico, the Rhône Delta, the North Sea, the Baltic Sea and the Adriatic Sea. Oxygen levels fall in these coastal waters. Dead Zone takes us on an eye-opening investigative journey across the globe, focussing on a dozen iconic species one-by-one and looking in each case at the role that industrial farming is playing in their plight.

This is a wake-up call for us all, laying bare the myths that prop up factory farming before exploring what we can do to save the planet with healthy food (Phillip Lymbery. 2017).

Desertification on 2/3 of the land on earth

Allan Savory. https://youtu.be/vpTHi7O66pI

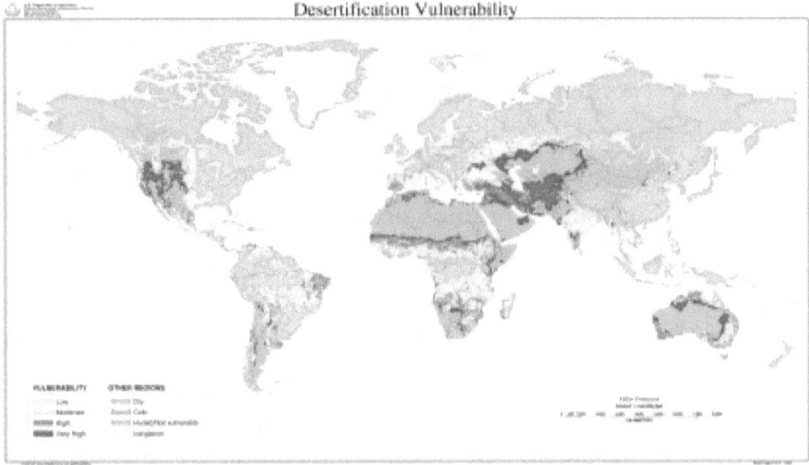

- When humans mastered fire, language and developed weapons like spears and axes, they were formidable predators. This was especially the case in the grasslands where their prey ran in herds. The grasslands with their deep, water and carbonaceous soils had developed for millions of years thanks to the balance between grazing animals, and the predators that fed with them.
- Modern farming methods contribute significantly to desertification and climate change due to water and air pollution from agriculture and intensive breeding of pigs, poultry and livestock. By breaking down agricultural land, we are reducing its enormous ability to retain and contain carbon.
- Chemical fertilizers to increase production have killed micro-

organisms in the soil, reduced fertility of the soil and the ability to retain water and led to additional flooding. Pesticides used for the treatment of internal parasites in animals have led to the destruction of dung beetles, which are vital for soil renewal.

- Fires break the ground cover in a way that it easily carries away by rain and wind. Huge man-made deserts have arisen. According NASA pictures from space about two thirds of the land is deserted.
- Banks finance the farmers to rent out their pastures for solar panels and windmills and to set up even more megafarms with the aid of electrical energy.

An ever-growing meat production causes drought and hunger in large parts of the world. Fast food and an increase in meat consumption in the West are also being imitated in other parts of the world. Modern agriculture makes an important contribution to desertification and climate change due to water and air pollution from agriculture and intensive breeding of pigs, poultry and livestock. By demolishing agricultural land, we reduce the enormous ability of land to hold carbon.

Wildlife loss

- In the last 50 years homo sapiens has wiped out 60% of mammals, birds, fish and reptiles in the wild
- Humankind has destroyed 83% of all mammals and half of plants since the dawn of civilization.
- Wildlife hunting in tropical forests reduces bird and mammal populations.

Our ancestors have likely consumed bushmeat, wild animals killed for food. During the 20th century, however, commercial hunting using firearms and wire snares to supply logging and oil exploration concessions along new roadway networks has dramatically increased the catch in Central African forests. Annually, it is estimated that 579 million wild animals are caught and consumed in the Congo basin, equaling 4.5 million tons of bushmeat, with the addition of a possible 5 million tons of wild mammalian meat from the Amazon basin. Tropical lowland forest habitat contains the world's greatest terrestrial biodiversity and may therefore harbor a reservoir of zoonotic pathogens. The wildlife trade in general generates in excess one billion direct and indirect contacts between humans and domesticated animals annually. The broad range of tissue and fluid exposures associated with the bush meat industry's hunting and butchering may take these wildlife interactions especially risky. In Africa, as many as 30 different species of primates are also hunted and processed by the bushmeat industry.

- The increase in meat products and dairy production in the West could only be achieved with artificial insemination of livestock and the animals unilaterally fattening with soy flour, corn and fish meal.
- One billion people suffer from hunger, while 70 billion

animals are fattened and eaten every year.

- During the ice ages the Cro-Magnon man was forced to eat more meat because there were fewer grains, fruit, nuts and seeds. Will modern man start eating more fruit and vegetables now that the earth is warming up?
- We can no longer ignore the impact of current unsustainable production models. If we start eating less meat, the farmers can gradually switch from intensive livestock farming to agriculture

Benítez-López A, Alkemade R, Schipper AM et al. The impact of hunting on tropical mammal and bird populations. Science 2017 356(6334):180-183

Population growth to seven, eight or nine billion causes food shortages, diseases and climate changes due to intensive meat production. The large number of animals locked up for meat consumption is the perfect system as a source for pathogenic viruses such as highly pathogenic influenza, corona virus and leukemia virus. The human race is moving in the same direction as the species that we have seen disappearing.

Downfall of Easter Island culture

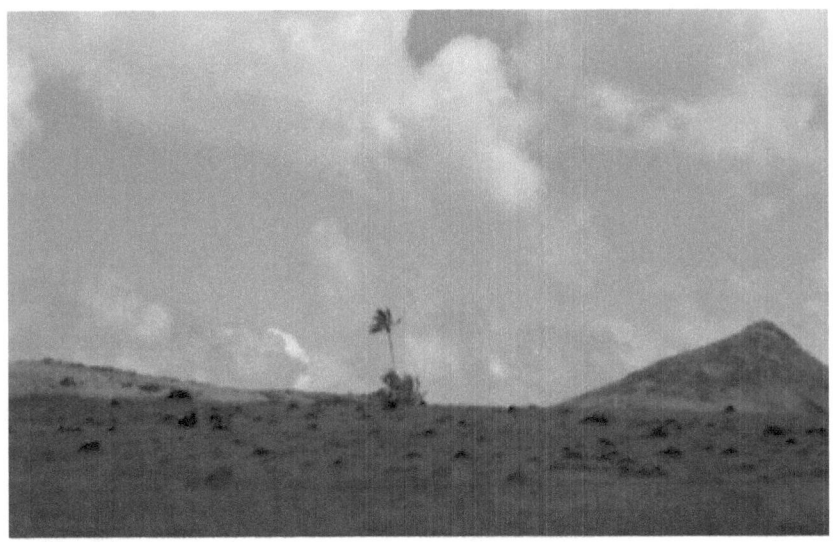

A last palmtree was left

- Along with the last trees, the birds and the raw materials for making spears and canoes were gone.
- Overpopulation and overexploitation of the increasingly scarce means put an end to the peaceful society after about 1,000 years and conflict and even cannibalism arose.

From Taiwan and Southeast China, three to four thousand years ago, the first brave seafarers with their double catamaran canoes with double sails, made from tree trunks and braided leaf fibers, explore the 10,000 volcanic islands in the Pacific. Thanks to their knowledge of wind, sea current and the stars, they have sailed further and further to the east. At the time of father Abraham, around 2,000 BC, these Chinese already reached New Guinea. Between 500 BC and 500 AD the island groups of the central Pacific were colonized. The big expeditions ended around 1,000 AD. The Polynesian triangle is located between Hawaii in the north, Tahiti and its islands in the west, New Zealand in the southwest and Easter Island in the East.

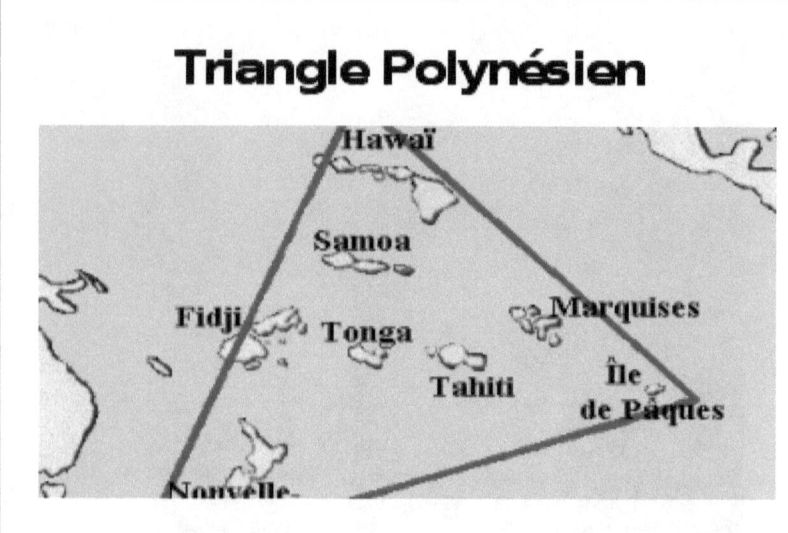

The inhabitants of the Polynesian triangle, the Maori of New Zealand, the Rapa Nui of Easter Island and the Hawaiians speak a related language. Residents of the Marquises Islands migrated from there to Easter Island. The Hawaiian Islands were between the years 500 and 700 conquered by these settlers. Easter Island has been as last about the year 700 discovered.

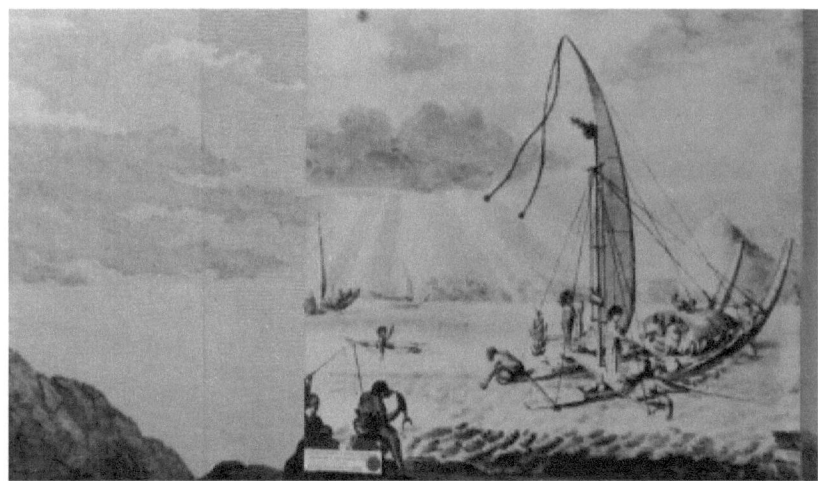

The history of man on Easter Island has started with a group of Polynesians from the Marquesas islands, around 400 AD have sailed to the east. They had brought all kinds of plants and seeds and the expedition was meant to colonize new land. Easter Island was about 700 AD discovered. New islands were found when birds were seen. Birds lay eggs on the land and their presence always means land in the neighborhood. More clouds over land are already visible from afar. These sailors also saw the pattern of the waves that an island had to be on their route. Easter Island lies 2,100 nautical miles (4,000 kilometers) after the Marquises Islands. Easter Island was uninhabited. The crater lakes in the three volcanoes contained drinking water and permanent establishment was therefore possible. They found a true paradise. The Polynesian settlers brought bananas, taro, sweet potato, sugar cane, paper mulberry, rats and chickens. The island was completely covered with palm trees. They found raw materials to make fabrics, cords and canoes. The birds in the forest, the fish from the ocean, the rats for the barbecue and the chickens provided the residents with food. The mild climate and fish-rich waters around the island gave the new residents a carefree life.

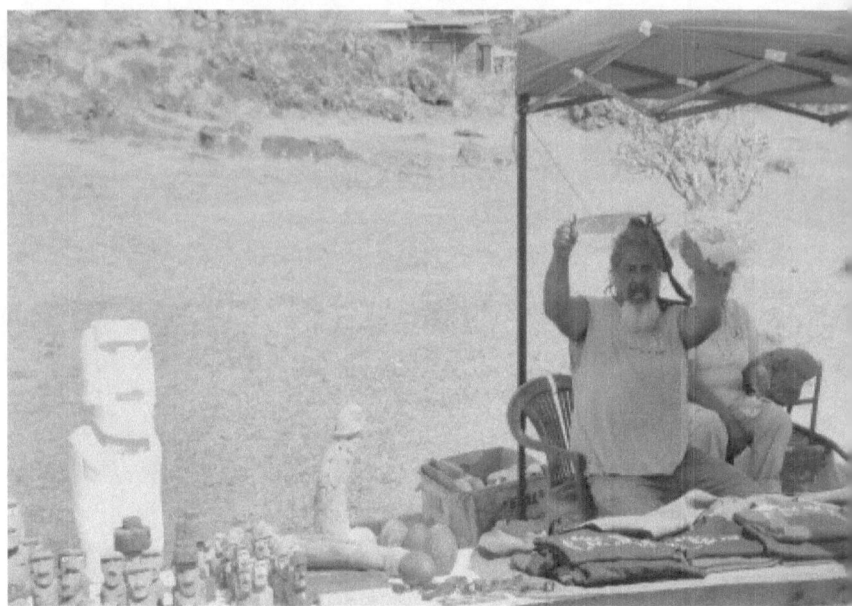

The Chinese origins of the Rapa Nui, the original inhabitants of the island, are still clearly recognizable

The population on the island grew rapidly, as a result of which increasingly larger parts of the forest were cut down. After all, ten groups lived on strips of land from the sea to the interior. The higher ranks lived on the coast with the holy places and the lower classes more inland. To thank the gods and to vote favorably, the inhabitants began to build the statues (or Moai) that make the island so famous. The Chinese culture has a very strong ancestor worship. These statues are representations of their forefathers, and the presence of such an image was seen as a kind of guardian angel for a village.

- **The European discovery of the island, by the navigator Jakob Roggeveen, took place in 1722**

On 1 August 1721, the then 62-year-old Jacob Roggeveen left with a fleet of the West India Company of the Reede van Texel. With three sailing ships they searched for "The Unknown Suydtland," a then suspected continent, which Roggeveen hoped to find with this expedition somewhere west of South America. New land, where trade posts could be thought of, could never be found. On Easter Sunday, April 5, 1722, an island was seen for the first time. They see smoke and fire and know that the island is inhabited. Since then, this island is called Easter Island.

- The island had been in complete isolation for 1,000 years by Polynesians, who never again undertook the 1,000 nautical miles journey back to the nearest land

Due to bad weather and heavy surf one could not land. On Wednesday, April 7, a small boat with a resident of Easter Island sailed towards their ships. They were met with a sloop. The indigenous man was forcibly brought on board De Arend and made a deep impression on Roggeveen and the crew. The next day Roggeveen went ashore with 134 crewmembers. Jacob Roggeveen was the first European to set foot on this small volcanic island in the Pacific Ocean. Some men felt threatened and began shooting against Roggeveen's explicit order. Twelve islanders were killed. As soon as the peace returned to Easter Island, an exploration of the island could be started. They studied the habits of the islanders and charted the island. According to Roggeveen's description, between two and three thousand people lived peacefully together on the island. With 170 square kilometers, Easter Island is the same size as the Dutch Wadden island of Texel, where Roggeveen had left.

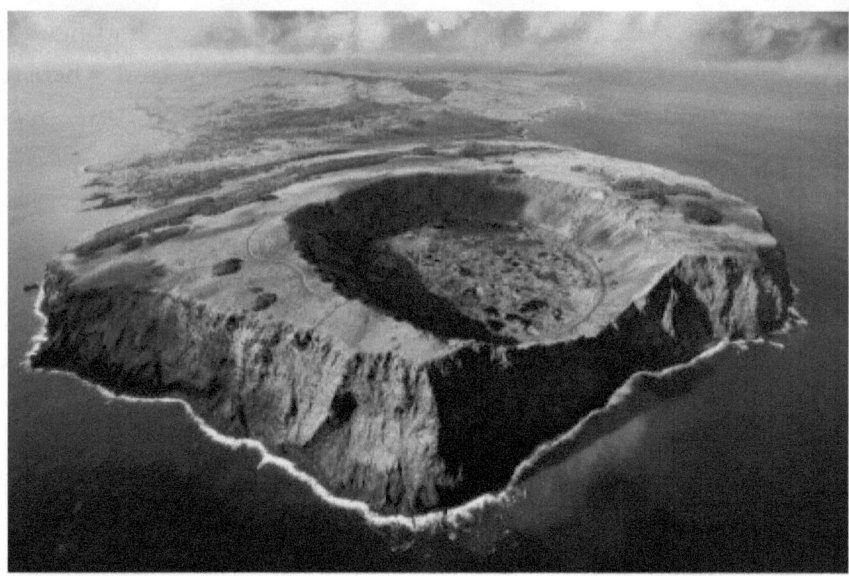

The Polynesians called their island "The Navel of the World" **(Te Pito O Te Henua).** Later, the name "Rapa Nui" means big rock, has become customary. At the time of Roggeveen the island was already bare and almost tree-less. Roggeveen counted about 2,000-3,000 inhabitants on the island, but it seems that there were 10,000-15,000 inhabitants in the 16th and 17th century.

Moai

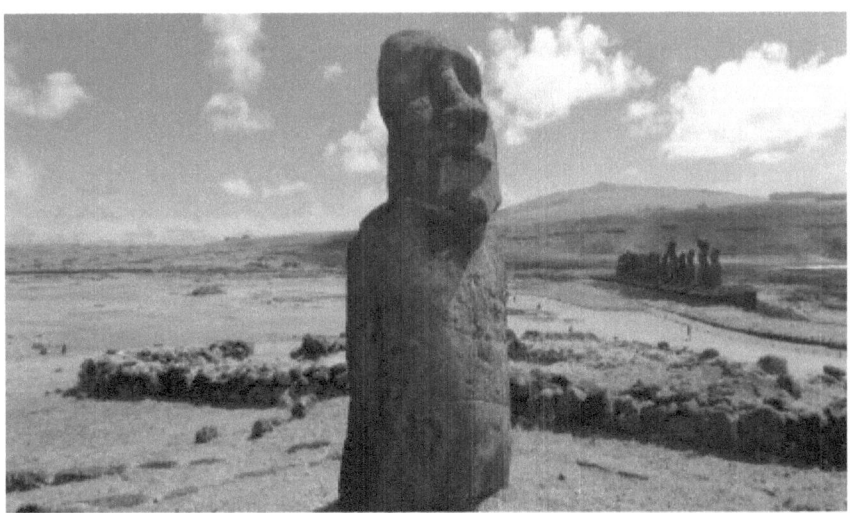

Most Moai were standing statues when Jakob Roggeveen arrived. Captain James Cook saw standing images as well as downed images when he landed on the island twenty years later in 1744. The last European mention of an upright statue was in 1838. Nothing was reported as standing in 1868.

According to traditions, the last statue that was overthrown was that of Paro (around 1840). In honor of her husband Paro was erected. This statue was almost 10 meters high and weighed 65 tons. Paro was brought down by enemies of the family and broken in the middle. In the 19th century, all standing statues were taken away during tribal wars, buried on their shoulders, to look like severed heads. The images were beaten down one by one intermittently by certain enemies of the owner of a statue, as described for Paro.

The end of civilization on Easter Island has little to do with environmental disasters, more with the arrival of the Spaniards, Italians and other Europeans. The original ancestor worship around the Moai was exchanged for imported Catholicism. Missionaries converted to faith the original population. In 1862 Peruvian ships captured more than a thousand residents to sell them as slaves to operators of guano mines along the Peruvian coast. New diseases brought by the Spaniards in the conquest of South America, such as smallpox and tuberculosis, have eradicated entire civilizations. Recurring Easter Islanders also brought deadly diseases. In 1877 the population of Easter Island was only 110 people. These 110 Rapanui had only 36 descendants, and they are the ancestors of all 2,296 Rapanui currently living on the island. The island was annexed by Chile in 1888, leaving around 4,000 Chileans on the island today. It has been determined by decree that only original residents, the Rapa Nui, may own land on the island.

Overpopulation

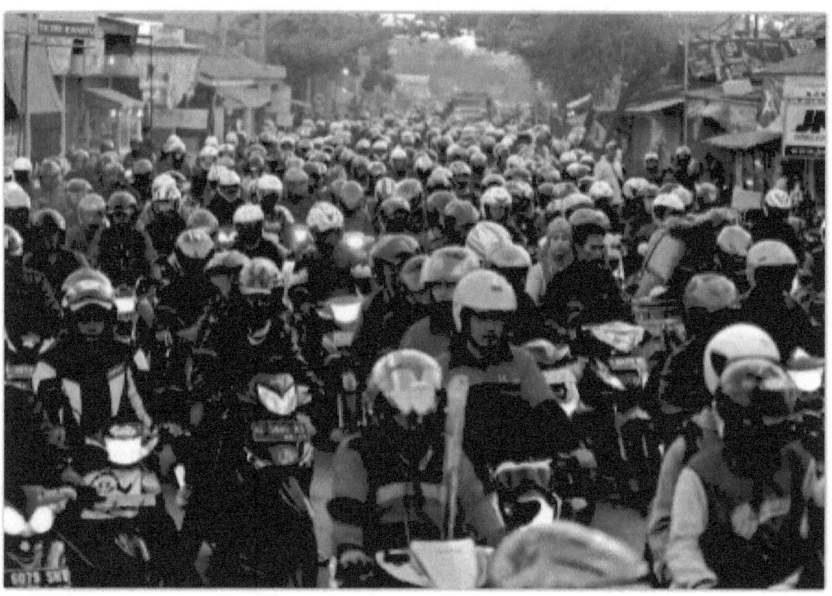

- For example, Indonesia. Half of the population is younger than 15 years.
- Young people take care of the elderly. Many children can take care of their retirement in the absence of a pension.
- When prosperity increased in Europe, the dependence on the elderly decreased and the population increase declined.
- Less prosperous countries can earn income by producing their own food with the new cultivation techniques.

In Singapore, the two-children policy began in the 1970s. Due to the enormous influx of immigrants, the population grew, but the indigenous population growth decreased. The one-child policy of China led to a population reduction of three hundred million people.

Countries with still extreme population growth are Brazil (fifty million inhabitants in 1950, more than two hundred ten million in

2018) and Indonesia (Java in 1960 sixty million inhabitants, one hundred and sixty million in 2018). Africa, now good for one fifth of the world's population, will be the only continent whose population will continue to grow after 2050. The UN expects that by 2100 40 percent of the world will be Africans.

- **If free contraception could be provided to women in Africa, who want to continue learning and work hard for more prosperity for their families, the increase in the population may also decrease here.**

The European population is shrinking. In Singapore, the two-child policy began in the 1970s. The population grew because of the enormous influx of immigrants, but the native population growth declined. China's one-child policy led to a population restriction of three hundred million people. Birth control is most common in China, with 83% of the population using one of the available contraceptives. Slightly less in Europe: 77% - and in North and South America 75%. In Africa, the percentage is shockingly low in some countries. Contraception is expected to increase by 2030 from 17 to 27 percent in West Africa, from 23 to 34 percent in Central Africa, from 40 to 55 percent in East Africa, and from 39 to 45 percent in Melanesia, Micronesia and Polynesia (Trends in contraceptive use worldwide, 2015 United Nations).

Primacy of the pharmaceutical industry

Many new cancer medicines do not heal, they sometimes even extend the life span for a short time, while they cost thousands of euros per month. These drugs are expensive because they can only be used in a small group of patients.

- Eribulin against metastatic breast cancer, costs € 145,000 per year of life gained and provides an average gain of 2.7 months life extension.
- Crizotinib, against non-small cell lung cancer, costs € 65,000 per year of life gained with an average gain of 4.7 months life extension.
- Abiraterone against metastatic prostate cancer, costs € 42,000 per year, with an average gain of 8 months of life.

The concept that cancer is a genetic disease, also infers that cancer development is irreversible because reversal of mutations back to a normal cell is extremely rare. The probability of mutating a normal cell to a cancer cell during cell division is approximate one in a million or so. If we assume the same probability for a back-mutation, the probability that a cell will become cancerous then reverse course is exceptionally low (probability is about one chance in a trillion). The assumption of the pharmaceutical industry that with surgery and radiotherapy incurable cancer only can be treated with medicines is fundamentally wrong. The pharmaceutical industry has made himself master to every facet of illness. No patient leaves the office without a prescription. The costs of cancer research and care exceed the benefits of the slight progression in cancer treatment and even of the five-year survival for the last 50 years. Since the fifties of the 20th century, intensive breeding in livestock has increased sharply. An increase that keeps pace with the recent increase in cancer mortality. Cancer is now number one cause of death.

There is a poignant shortage in education in nutritional science among cancer researchers and clinicians. Prevention is preferable to cure. The pharmaceutical industry only develops and sells medicines that make money. The industry is now feverishly looking for the anti-aging pill. That is not to blame commercial companies. Well-functioning first generation antibiotics, painkillers, antihypertensive drugs etc. are replaced by newer drugs if the patents have expired.

The oldest and cheapest antibiotic

In 1980, anthropologist George Armelagos and medical analyst Mark Nelson of Paratek Pharmaceuticals discovered traces of the antibiotic tetracycline in human bones from 350 - 550 AD. Tetracycline is produced by streptomyces, a bacterium that is often found on grain. When fermenting grain to make beer, streptomyces produces large amounts of the antibiotic. It is therefore not surprising that tetracycline was found in the bones of the people of that time. In more recent research on the bones, Armelagos and Nelson discovered that the bones were saturated with it. Apparently the Nubians deliberately produced the antibiotic for the treatment of diseases. Even in the bones of very young children died, the substance was found in large quantities. An indication that the beer foam was prescribed to sick children. We always assumed that the discovery of tetracycline did not take place until 1948. Streptomyces grows in a gold colony that floated on top of the beer. It is possible that this golden color also had an important meaning for the Nubians.

Favorable results of combined therapy of azithromycin with the chemotherapy on non-small cell lung cancer patients

Although new chemotherapeutic drugs have been applied constantly, their efficacy for non-small cell lung cancer (NSCLC) is still not satisfactory. In recent years, epidemiological investigations have shown that lung cancer may be induced by chronic Chlamydia pneumonia (Cpn) infection. This study (Chu DJ 2014) of azithromycin, commonly used for the treatment of Cp infections, combined with the chemotherapeutics paclitaxe and cisplatin on stage III-IV NSCLC patients achieved favorable results in terms of side effects and overall survival.

Azithromycin, a macrolide antibiotic as well as erythromycin, prevents bacteria from growing by interfering with their protein synthesis. It binds to the bacterial ribosome, thereby inhibiting the translation of mRNA and protein synthesis.

The afore mentioned examinations and treatments have been applied with favorable results by treating physicians with longer existing drugs whose patents had long expired. These experiments deserve to be copied and would greatly reduce the costs of medical treatments and could open a new treatment trail apart from the double-blind search of the pharmaceutical industry for better and more profitable drugs. My previously suggested idea of treating lung cancer with previous infections with Chlamydiae for a long time with doxycycline (a derivative form of tetracycline) can also have a favorable result.

Co-therapy with tetracycline and azithromycin (Ferreri AJ)

Malignant lymphomas were treated with tetracycline (doxycycline) and their disappearance was similar to eradication of the Chlamydia bacteria detected in the cells (Ferreri AJ 2005). Tetracycline and macrolide (erythromycin) antibiotics have a striking therapeutic effect on Chlamydia infection. Cp infection can be controlled and prevented. Penicillin kills bacteria by preventing the bacteria from rebuilding their cell wall after division. Chlamydiae have no cell wall and, like viruses, are completely dependent on their host cells. Once in the host cell, Chlamydiae are not susceptible to penicillin. Tetracyclines prevent these cell parasites from using the metabolic processes of the host cell. Chlamydiae need these to form new proteins for growth and multiplication. Tetracycline is produced from chlortetracycline, a compound derived from Streptomyces aureofaciens. Tetracyclines are able to enter the host cells of the Chlamydiae through the pores of the cell wall. Once inside the cell, tetracycline causes inhibition of DNA and protein synthesis that these cell parasites need for their own growth and multiplication.

The next stage in evolution

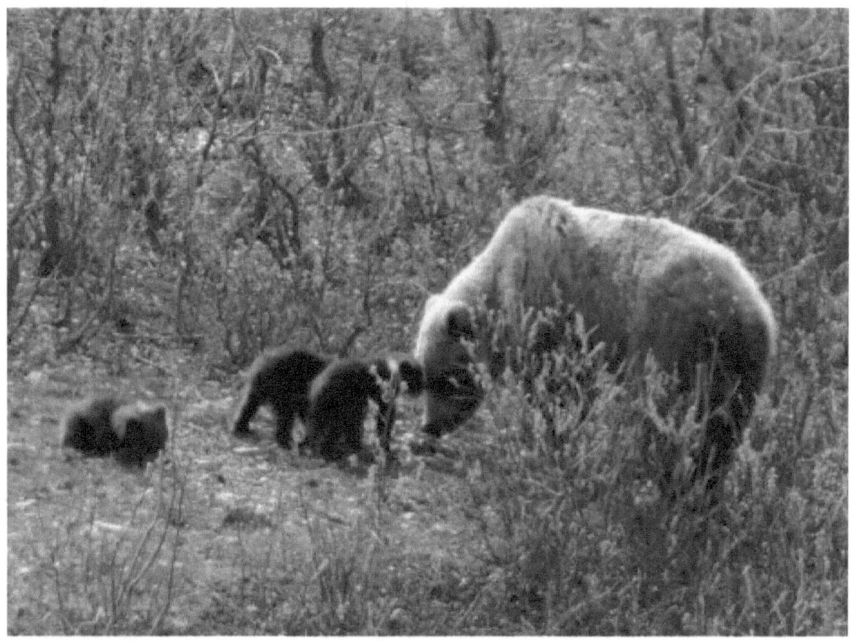

Boar with three youngs in Denali tundra wilderness

All mammals must have the opportunity to care for their offspring themselves.

Artificial insemination of livestock and factory farming of cows, goats, pigs, sheep and rabbits is a gross violation of this fundamental mammalian right.

"Nothing will benefit human health anymore and increase the chance of survival on earth as much as the evolution towards a vegetarian diet."

- Albert Einstein

Grasslands and grazing animals have an enormous ability to hold carbon. Agriculture can produce better vegetable and fruit as food for humans than the corn and soybeans with which we now fatten and confine the animals in factory farms to be eaten by humans.

Man, the most intelligent mammal, also has a natural urge to care for their offspring, which unfortunately is often violated by an increasing number of divorces. It will take 18 years for the child to become independent as an adult. Before the time of the birth control pill, it was a great shame for family and fellow believers to have a child as unmarried ones and the mother often had to give up the child. Penetrating sexuality and conceiving children were exclusively intended for marriage. Until the marriage, the mature woman had to remain a virgin. Once married, it was important to remain faithful until death do us part to get a place in heaven. The voluntary celibacy of laymen offered some guarantee for a close-knit family and religious life.

Buddhists, Hindus and Augustine as a trendsetter for Christians had no knowledge of the possibilities for humans to travel to the moon and beyond into the sky and for women to be free from the instinctive process of reproduction.

Marriages are increasingly closed in the 21st century if one or more children are already conceived. There are fewer ecclesiastical blessings. There are even blind date marriages. In the interest of the child, a more binding agreement is desperately needed. Why not every marriage to be concluded by a notary who at the same time draws up a civil contract for the couple, male and female, or as is the case today with the same sex. The agreement may state that the marriage cannot be dissolved until the last child conceived is 18 years old and the accommodation of both partners is arranged.

How not to die and stay healthy

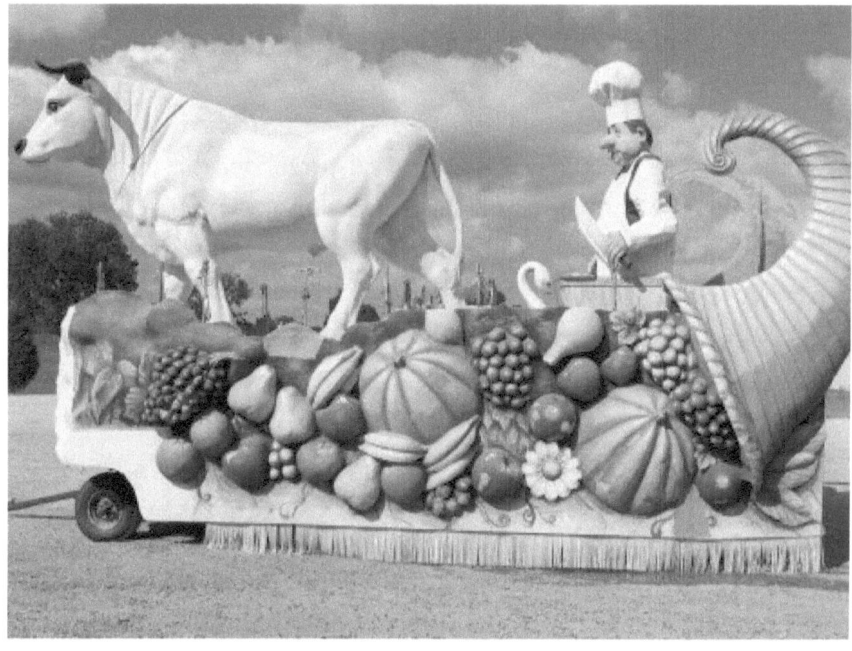

How to become healthy 100 years old

We eat everything that tastes good. If it is cheap and tasty, it also accelerates chronic disease and tumor formation. This is how our food system works. The raw materials for factory preparation are limited. Soy, corn, eggs, refined sugars, animal proteins and trans fats. These are the main ingredients that the largest food companies use to make the food that is all around us. It is not that these big companies do not care. In fact, it is difficult for them to do something else. In parts of the world with less chemical agriculture, less factory food processing, mortality from cancer is lower. Fruits and vegetables contain more bio-active substances.

- Fruits and vegetables make bio-active substances that delay the growth and propagation of intruders.

Plant-based nutrition works life-extending

Voluntary restriction of the diet will probably never gain much popularity as a life-prolonging strategy. Vegetable diets have a low methionine content. Vegetable proteins - especially those from vegetables or nuts - contain less methionine than animal proteins. Several animal studies with methionine restricted diet have shown inhibition of cancer cell growth and prolonged healthy life span in experimental animals. American researchers have looked at 30 years of nutrition data among 130,000 people. They found a reduced risk of premature death in those who ate more vegetable protein and a higher risk in those who ate more animal protein. Each increase of 3% more vegetable proteins in the diet reduced the risk of death, by whatever cause, during the period under review by 10%. A link was also shown with a 12% lower risk of death from cardiovascular disease. But a 10% higher share of animal proteins in the diet led to a 2% higher risk of death and 8% higher chance of dying of a heart problem (Song M).

Plant-based food is not boring and one-sided. Exotic fruits, herbs, soya and vegetables can very well replace all meat and meat products in our supermarkets. On the land, 250,000 different varieties of plants can be grown and in oceans there are another 20,000 different species, including seaweed, rich in omega-3 oils. The countries of the southern hemisphere could also make a larger contribution to this. The recipe is still in its infancy.

Animal proteins and vegetable proteins from the oceans are healthier than animal proteins from intensive livestock farming. The oceans offer a good choice of anchovies, mussels, oysters, squid, herring, mackerel, cod, sprat, sole, crabs, lobsters, shrimps and even wild tuna and salmon.

The human body defends against invading bacteria, spores and yeast cells, with the help of antibodies, white blood cells, macrophages and T-cells. The body is unable to produce antioxidants such as beta-carotene, vitamin C and is unable to make vegetable bio-active substances.

Unnatural nutrition is the cause of deficits and chronic diseases. Fast food, many meat products and little fruit and vegetables weaken the natural defenses. The question remains how a revolution in public opinion can be achieved in order to massively switch exclusively to natural food with supplementing necessary supplements for existing shortages.

Vitamin C

Not so long ago during the great voyages of discovery, it has already been discovered that vitamin C deficiencies arise due to lack of fresh fruit and vegetables. This gave the sailors scurvy with internal bleeding, which usually resulted in death. Vitamin C is necessary for the construction of connective tissue proteins. Deficient production of these connective tissue proteins weakens the blood vessels with bleeding as a result. Due to the frequent use of pesticides in agriculture, the content of bioactive antibodies in fruit and vegetables has been reduced, as a result of which our defense against cell infections is even more affected.

Vitamin D

Sufficient vitamin D increases bone density, which means less chance of bone fractures. Vitamin D is not really a vitamin, but the precursor of the powerful steroid hormone calcitrol, which has widespread actions throughout the body. Several studies have shown that vitamin D deficiency increases the risk of developing cancer and that avoiding a deficiency and adding vitamin D supplements can be an economical and safe way to reduce the incidence of cancer and the prognosis and result of cancer treatment. Vitamin D is a fat-soluble vitamin and is sold as pearl capsules. Vitamin supra D3 forte capsules (Bayer) contain 20 mcg equivalent to 800 IU. If a deficiency has been established, at least 2 pearls per day should be taken.

Coconut fat

Coconut oil is a vegetable fat that is well processed by the body. The grease already melts at a temperature of 24 degrees Celsius and is resistant to high temperatures. Coconut fat is very suitable for baking and roasting. One or two coffee spoons (5-10 ml) is sufficient. When firing for frying and roasting, less combustion products form than when heating the other vegetable oils, sunflower oil and olive oil. It promotes the absorption of the fat-soluble vitamins A-D-E and K. Vegetable fat contains nutrients for nerve and brain cells. Overweight and diabetes mellitus are common in later life. For these risk groups it has been demonstrated that the use of 40 ml coconut fat per day has a beneficial effect. When the body produces too little insulin, the energy supply (glucose) to the brain is jeopardized. Coconut fat promotes an alternative energy supply to the brain cells after admission. Coconut oil has a beneficial effect on the energy intake of brain cells and memory loss in Alzheimer's disease (De la Rubia Orti 2017).

Curcuma

Curcuma, a natural polyphenol compound, isolated from the rhizome of a herbaceous perennial plant, has anticancer activity. We need to consume a sufficient amount of bio-active substances with fruit and vegetables to keep out invaders. Bioactive antibodies inhibit the overactivity of the enzyme CYP1B1 in cancer cells. Infected or damaged cells are now seen as abnormal and are removed from the body by growth inhibition and the death of the infected cell.

Benefits of Mediterranean food

The diet in Spain, Italy and Greece is one of the healthiest eating habits in the world. There are apparently fewer diseases here, and mortality from some chronic diseases is also less. This dietary pattern is rich in fruit and vegetables, fish and less saturated fat containing dairy products. This eating habit reduces the risk of cardiovascular disease, reduces the risk of diabetes, prolongs the lifespan and counts more healthy elderly people.

Avoid fast food and unhealthy trans fats

Old McDonald's farm is very different than the McDonald of today. Fast food is in fashion. Hamburgers and chicken burgers are often on the menu of hard-working people. It is no longer rare for someone to go to bed with a bag of chips.

Vegetable (unsaturated) fats are liquid at room temperature and can only be processed by the food industry as a solid substance. These fats are converted into partially hardened fat by a chemical process. Products that contain partially hydrogenated fats and trans fatty acids, such as margarine, chips, cookies, coffee milk powder, tarts, crackers and pizzas are bad for blood vessels. Nowadays, croissants are often made with hydrogenated vegetable oils instead of butter. Cheap mass production means that a croissant contains more fat (17 grams), which consists of about one third (5 to 6 grams) of trans fats.

It is difficult and often impossible to escape the temptations of major industrial interests.

- Light products are the answer of the sugar industry. Fats are replaced by sugars by the food industry, which has a counterproductive effect and makes us eat more.

How to stay healthy

* no colds
    * don't smoke
    * with clean indoor air, don't keep birds in home
    * wash hands regularly
    * eat more vegetable proteins
    * do not eat animals
    * train for one hour three times a week

So you become a hundred years
    * do not fall
    * do not have an accident
    * don't get a cold
    * do not choke, pneumonia most common cause of death for centenarians

How Not to Die

The vast majority of premature deaths can be prevented through changes in diet and lifestyle. In How Not to Die, Dr. Michael Greger, examines the fifteen top causes of premature death in America - heart disease, various cancers, diabetes, Parkinson's, high blood pressure, and more - and explains how nutritional and lifestyle interventions can sometimes trump prescription pills and other pharmaceutical and surgical approaches, freeing us to live healthier lives.

How Not to Die. Gene Stone & Michael Greger, MD

The China Study was a detailed study about the connection between nutrition and heart disease, diabetes, and cancer. The report also examines the source of nutritional confusion produced by powerful lobbies, government entities and opportunistic scientists. The China Study observed in rural China and Taiwan whether there were patterns of associations for different dietary, lifestyle and disease characteristics within the survey of 65 counties, 130 villages and 6,500 adults and their families. Among the many associations that are relevant to diet and disease, so many pointed to the same finding: people who ate the most animal-based foods got the most chronic disease. Even relatively small intakes of animal-based foods were associated with adverse effects. People who ate the most plant-based foods were the healthiest and tended to avoid chronic disease.

The China Study. Campbell TC, PhD, **Campbell TM,** MD (2006)

Simply make your own meals

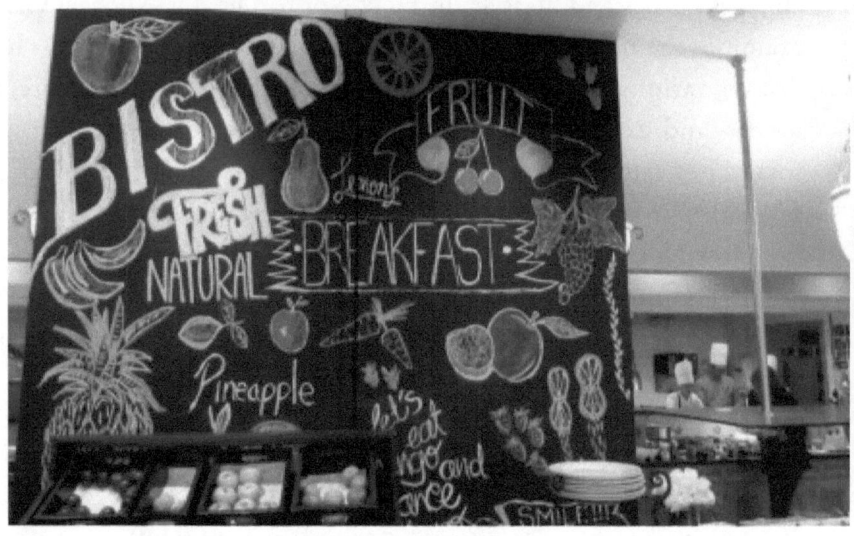

Stick to this simple advice to get rid of excess body fat and prevent diseases. Only little whole meal bread, pasta and rice to lose weight faster. Nutrition must contain many vegetables, but also sufficient vegetable proteins and fats (fish, olive oil, avocado, etc.).

Start with a plant-based diet, and the need for animal proteins and fats will gradually decline

In addition to diet, physical activity and extra antioxidant intake may counteract DNA methylation changes contributing to aging.

Fruit Breakfast

Start with two glasses of water

Oatmeal flakes with broken flax seed in soy yoghurt or soya light, almond milk or coconut milk, with fresh fruit. Like strawberries, raspberries, apples, pear, mandarin, orange, melon etc. Cut the fruit into pieces to preserve the dietary fiber.

Soup with the lunch

Make soup from vegetable broth. Think of tomato, vegetable, onion, pumpkin, mushroom, broccoli soup. A delicious soup can be made of all vegetables.

Salad with nuts, mushrooms, arugula, tomato, onion, garlic, green beans, kidney beans, chickpeas etc. Olive oil dressing.

Sandwich with salad of tuna, salmon, shrimp etc. or an omelet or hardboiled egg. Omega-3 rich fish such as salmon, herring, mackerel and shellfish like mussels are much healthier than red meat.

- *No sausages, hard-boiled eggs only, no meat (products) from the super, no insufficiently cooked BBQ meat, less dairy products, no raw milk cheese.*

Hot meal

Make especially use of herbs and spices. Replace the meat you were used to for example with chickpeas, brown or white beans. Make a delicious chili sin carne or curry dish with cauliflower, broccoli and chickpeas.

Bake and roast with coconut fat or olive oil

Coconut fat is very suitable for baking and roasting. Melt a coffee spoon (5 ml) in the pan is sufficient. When heating and roasting, less combustion products form than when heating the other vegetable oils, sunflower oil and olive oil.

No dessert

Avoid in case of excess weight sugars and quickly digestible carbohydrates. More healthy fats give a feeling of satiety and forces the liver to burn absorbed fats and belly fats when energy is required by the body. By sweetening, the liver chooses the path of least resistance (glycolysis) and provides the requested energy, glucose, and stores excess to body fat.

Drink black coffee, green tea or ginger tea after the meal. Ginger tea can be made by cutting slices from ginger root and letting it boil in boiling water.

Olives, nuts.

- *Alcohol and wine in moderation. The degradation product acetaldehyde is harmful to our DNA. Too many wine acids damage the esophagus and stomach.*

Your Target Weight

The abdominal circumference around the navel in relation to body height is a good measure of (over) weight. Belt length 93 cm divided by body length 186 cm = 0.5 should preferably be less than 50%

Men	Women	
< 35%	< 35%	Underweight
35% - 45%	35% - 42%	Extremely Slim
43% - 46%	42% - 46%	Healthy
46%– 53%	46% - 49%	Normal Weight
53% - 58%	49% - 54%	Overweight
58% - 63%	54% - 58%	Obese
> 63%	> 58%	Highly Obese

Burning Belly Fat

Fat burning only starts after twenty minutes of exercise. Until this time of 20 minutes, especially carbohydrate reserves (the glycogen in the liver and muscles) are burned and you will not lose weight. This means that you start the fat burning process during the last part of the training. That is why it is better to exercise for one hour three times a week (3 x 40 minutes fat burning) than six times a week for half an hour (6 x 10 minutes fat burning). It does not matter what the training consists of. This can be brisk walking, slow jogging or a session on a treadmill or rowing machine.

Hydrogen, energy to the future

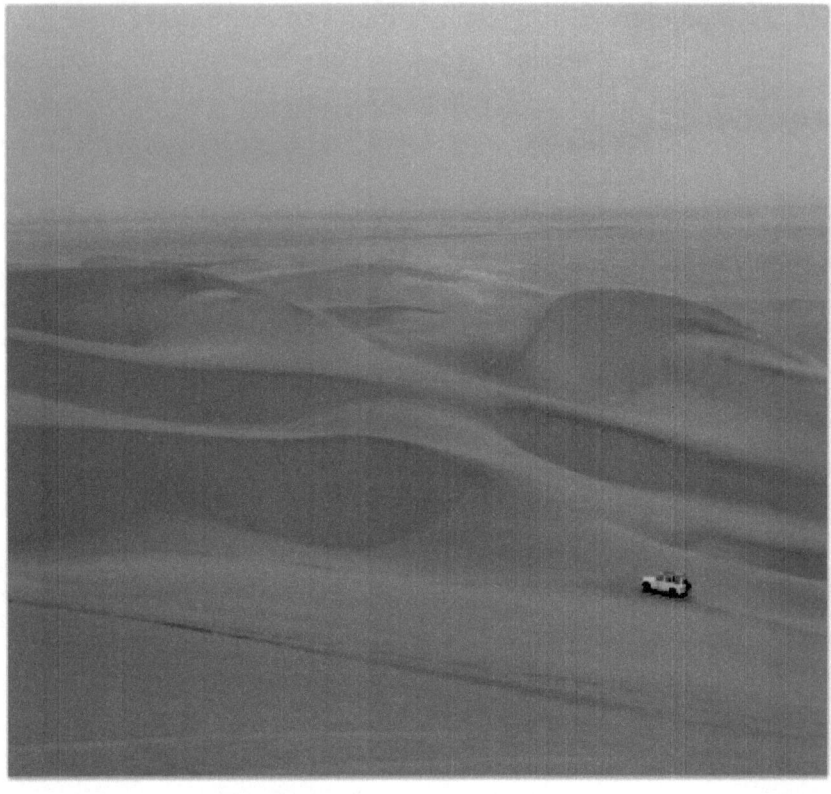

The Namib desert at Lüderitz, a port on the Atlantic Ocean on the south-west coast of Namibia, is one of the sunniest places in the world. This desert is 200 km wide and extends 2000 km from Angola in the North to the Orange River in the South along the Atlantic Ocean. In this 81,000 km2 a suitable area for energy production can be found. A combination of solar panels and hydrogen gas production with transport to the sea can offer economic benefits to poor Namibia. https://youtu.be/a04JKguARZA

In 54 minutes, drops to the earth the amount of solar energy that the whole world consumes in one year. All free renewable energy. Only it is in the wrong place at the wrong time in the wrong form. If we turn all that energy into hydrogen on a daily basis, the scarcity of energy is immediately over. All this energy can be stored in the form of hydrogen and transported through the gas network and in liquid form by ship. Every day that we do nothing with the storage of solar and wind energy here and there in the Netherlands and in the deserts is a lost day. It's not really complicated, we just have to make the right decisions.

We will be saying goodbye not only to fossil fuels, but also to biofuels. The demand for palm oil has risen so much what is largely due to western policy to stimulate the use of biofuels. The cosmetics and food industries are also major customers. Fires has become increasingly fierce in recent years in the Brazilian Amazon forest and in the Indonesian tropical rainforests of Borneo and Papua New Guinea. The 'slash and burn' method (felling and burning) is used to cultivate natural land for palm plantations. Hydrogen as prime energy source is the solution.

- Let Groningen earn from the transition to hydrogen gas. The Netherlands already has an extensive gas network from Groningen to the rest of the Netherlands. This natural gas network can be used for hydrogen gas transport without too much adaptation so that most domestic and industrial connections can use hydrogen gas for heating, cooking and industrial use.
- Veendam has the first larger hydrogen plant in the Netherlands that uses solar power. It is an important step in Groningen's mission to develop into the hydrogen province of the Netherlands. Renewable energy from the electricity grid and 5,000 solar panels on the site provide green electricity to the plant, which can convert one megawatt of sustainable electricity into hydrogen. A hydrogen industry in Groningen can supply the large amounts of energy that will

be lost when the oil and gas era is closed. Hydrogen can be stored in empty salt caverns on the EnergyStock site. If all the salt caverns on the site are filled with hydrogen, that will be enough to heat all the houses in the Netherlands for several weeks.

- Researchers from the University of Waterloo in Canada have developed a new fuel cell that lasts at least ten times longer than current technology. These fuel cells can produce electricity from the chemical reaction, when hydrogen and oxygen are combined to make water, and will therefore be much cheaper. If these fuel cells are mass-produced, they will be able to power hydrogen-gas hybrid vehicles. http://www.uwaterloo.ca

- Canadian engineers have found a way to produce hydrogen relatively easily and cheaply. By injecting oxygen into the tar sands, the temperature in the soil appears to rise. As a result, hydrogen gas is released from the oil, which can be separated from other gases by special membrane filters. The procedure works in tar sands, but also exhausted and discarded oil fields: wherever there is still oil in the ground that can be heated, leading to the formation of hydrogen gas. Even with oil fields that are still in use, this technique can be used. A polluting fossil resource can thus be given a new lease of life and produce the energy carrier of the future. Hydrogen production is a cost-effective alternative to energy production from oil fields and tar sands. By placing hydrogen filter membranes in the production sources, only the hydrogen is extracted and undesirable by-products such as carbon dioxide diode and methane remain in the soil.

- The existing infrastructure and distribution channels around the oil fields would suffice, keeping production costs low. At the moment it costs about 2 dollars to produce a kilo of H2, but with the new method that would only be 10 to 50 cents. The necessary oxygen can be produced on site. This requires no more than 5 percent of the energy produced.

- The oil sands deposits in Western Canada not only represent a vast store of hydrocarbons (oil) that can be converted into fuel and petrochemicals but also a vast hydrogen store – a super clean valuable energy vector and chemical feedstock. Oil sands reservoirs have low energy and emissions intensities, hydrogen production is a viable alternative for energy production from heavy oil and oil sands reservoirs by using in situ gasification technology. Gasification reactions, together with the water-gas shift reaction, enable the generation of hydrogen from both bitumen and water within the oil sands reservoir. With hydrogen separation membranes in the production wells, other products from the reactions remain in the reservoir.

- Researchers at the Lawrence Berkeley National Laboratory (LBL) in California have developed a new type of solar cell. It is a so-called hybrid photovoltaic cell that can produce both electricity and hydrogen. These solar panels convert electricity that has not been taken from them into hydrogen during the day and store it. After all, a fuel cell can be used to convert hydrogen into electricity in the hours when there is no sunlight or when there is a very high demand, as a back-up. The HPEV solar panels (Hybrid Photo Electrochemical and Voltaic) increase efficiency in the generation and use of green electricity and can therefore contribute to achieving a lower price for green hydrogen. This is one of the biggest challenges at the moment, because the production of hydrogen from natural gas is even much cheaper. The HPEV-panels also have a third electrode for converting CO2. The

HPEV-panels have a third electrode, which uses the maximum possible number of electrons to generate hydrogen. The other two electrodes are used to generate electricity, just like conventional solar panels. The researchers are investigating whether this technology could also be used, for example, to remove CO_2 from the air and convert it into usable chemical applications. In any case, it seems that a new type of solar panel is in the making.

- In Stad aan het Haringvliet, The Netherlands, houses are being built with a system for storing solar energy in green hydrogen. This creates the entire chain of sustainable and renewable energy production, storage and use in the living environment. The solar energy from the summer period is stored for use in the winter months (seasonal storage). The gas network of the village can be switched to hydrogen with little cost and inconvenience for residents. The fifteen-kilometer gas network at Stad aan 't Haringvliet is flushed with nitrogen to remove natural gas. `The four gas district stations will be adjusted and the gas pipes in the homes will be checked. The natural gas central heating boilers are replaced by a hydrogen boiler. www.solencopower.com[1]

- The houses are completely self-sufficient in terms of energy requirements. Unique and the future of new constructions.

Chemical preparation of hydrogen from sodium borohydride
Sodium boron hydride (NaBH 4) is a chemical compound from which hydrogen can be extracted. In combination with fuel cells, electricity can be produced safely and with only water as a residual product. The material is a white powder and a well-known ingredient of washing powders. A Dutch inventor brought sodium boron hydride into contact with very pure water and a catalyst. The result: more

---

1. http://www.solencopower.com

than 95% of the theoretically feasible amount of hydrogen is actually extracted. A great success that has since been patented and is being further developed, in collaboration with Technical University Delft. You do need water without ions. It is transported to the filling station in granular form. A machine there makes ultrapure water from tapwater. The ultrapure water is then mixed with the sodium boron hydride, creating a pumpable slurry. The 'slurry' - called H2Fuel - is then filled up, just like you fill up with petrol. However, while you're doing that, you're also filling up with highly diluted hydrochloric acid. This is stored in a separate tank from the H2Fuel. If you want to drive, that hydrochloric acid is mixed with the H2Fuel and hydrogen is released within milliseconds. Not only from the sodium boron hydride, but also from the ultrapure water. The hydrogen then goes to the fuel cell, generating electricity. The reaction also results in a number of residual products, including water from the fuel cell. Some of it is filtered back into ultrapure water and used immediately, because you need more of this water than you can fill up with.

A truck, with only 350 liters of sodium boron hydride can go up and down to Barcelona without refueling. H2Fuel could also be the solution for storing excess renewable energy (generated by solar panels on sunny days, for example) for days with energy shortages (when it is very cloudy or windless, for example). H2Fuel can then help. But if you're going to refuel later, you'll have to leave the residual products behind. This means that truckers have to drive back and forth: they have to bring sodium boron hydride and dispose of residual products. From a logistical point of view, this is much more complicated and therefore more expensive. In addition, H2Fuel requires considerable modification of the existing (hydrogen) car. After all, you have to have three tanks: one for the sodium boron hydride, one for the diluted hydrochloric acid and one for the spent fuel. The company creates these three tanks by placing partitions in a tank and expects the automotive industry to implement this tank in the near future, but that is still questionable.

- The H2Fuel process, with a very high yield, has already been validated by TNO (www.h2-fuel.nl[2]). Hydrogen gas is not extracted from the ground and can be produced anywhere in the world (www.h2fuel.com[3]).
- H2Fuel, a sodium-borohydride compound, is the carrier of hydrogen. The chemical name is NaBH4 (powder) and can be stored indefinitely under normal atmospheric conditions. To release the hydrogen, Ultra Pure Water (UPW = fully pure H2O) and a little dilute hydrochloric acid are added in a certain ratio and the hydrogen molecules of both the NaBH4 and H2O are released. A total of 8H. This high yield of hydrogen molecules is only possible with the use of UPW (patented). With this hydrogen, electricity and / or heat can be produced via a fuel cell.
- NaBH4 + 2 H2O = 4 H2 + NaBO2 + heat. The residual product NaBO2 can be converted into NaBH4 in a new chemical process. The energy required for this can be supplied by solar and / or wind energy. The average power of a Dutch windmill is around 1,000 kWh.
- H2Fuel is completely free from any harmful emissions during production, storage, transport and consumption. The environmental tax can then expire in the long term.
- On sea-going vessels osmosis allows UPW to extract fully pure water from seawater and space is available for this type of power plant.
- A grant project to speed up the chemical preparation of hydrogen would be great. A greenhouse complex in the

2. http://www.h2-fuel.nl

3. http://www.h2fuel.com

Westland wants to be able to produce energy-neutral fruit and vegetables all year round with the help of a hydrogen power plant. Some vans are also converted into hydrogen cars and can refuel at the greenhouse complex and have the residual liquid here upgraded.

- Vertical agriculture and horticulture require a lot of heat, light and space to produce strawberries, lettuce, cauliflower, peppers, grapes and also tropical fruit such as pineapples all year round. Here too, such a power plant with fuel cells can be used. Farmers can give their warehouses a new destination. With local production with a greater supply and diversity, the current supply of fruit and vegetables over the equator will be able to decrease.

The hydrogen route within long-distance and heavy transport, heating and heavy industry will be at the forefront of cost reduction. A global scaling up of hydrogen applications is the most important contribution to a lower price. It starts at the hydrogen production process will become considerably more efficient. The substantial expansion of the tank infrastructure will reduce distribution and refueling costs sharply.

Vertical farming

Vertical farming, multilayer cultivation, is also called city farming

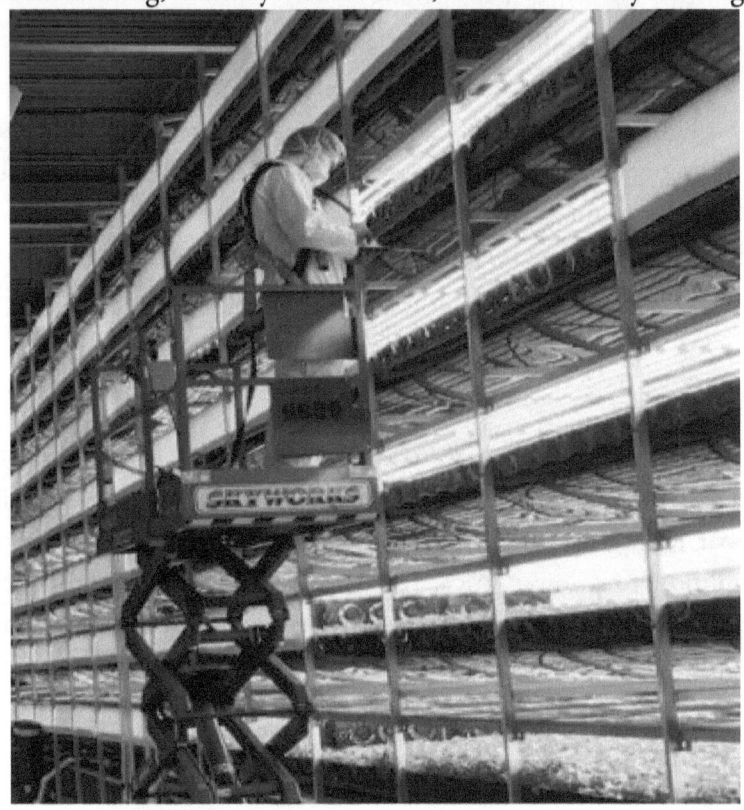

The usual agriculture and horticulture run on artificial fertilizers, pesticides and new plant varieties

- Unsprayed fruit and vegetables, pesticides are no longer needed
- In such a closed system, pests and diseases are no longer a chance

- Growing in two weeks which takes 30 days in the open ground with 95 percent less water consumption, fewer fertilizers, and completely without pesticides.
- Techniques can also be applied outside Europe and the USA.

Sunlight cannot be controlled. And the high-pressure sodium lamps with which Dutch growers provide extra light for their greenhouses can only be used to a limited extent. They give orange / yellow light and are too warm to place near plants. With the cooler LED lamps, which can contain all kinds of colors, engineers can develop a light recipe. They can choose the right combinations of wavelengths and light intensities, place the LED lamps near the plants, and opt for wider or narrower light beams. By altering the color of lights change the smell, taste and even the vitamin content of tomatoes. For more efficient growth, switch on the red light; to develop shorter plants with higher levels of antioxidants, use more blue light.

The reason for the higher yield, compared to greenhouses and outdoor cultivation, is that under LED lighting the entire plant, the whole year and long days can get enough light. In the uncontrolled sunlight, moreover, part is lost because one sheet gets too much and the other gets too little. Light is also lost due to reflection and the falling of photons on the ground. In order to make the collection of light more efficient, companies can drop light beams onto the leaves at certain angles. Or place LED lamps between plants. Strawberries are sweeter and tastier when the leaves and fruit are extra lighted. Dozens of vertical farms, also called 'vegetable factories' or 'indoor farms', supply spinach, bok choy, dill or cabbage every day. In climate-controlled rooms grow in four layers among others grow lettuce, strawberries, coriander and watercress. In an average Dutch greenhouse, the lettuce yield is 60 kilos per square meter of floor per year. 100 kilograms per square meter shelf will be taken in the vertical shelves. In Miyagi, Japan, a Japanese plant physiologist ordered 17,500

LED lamps that had to be installed in a former Sony factory. This factory supplies 10,000 unsprayed lettuce heads per day. In Singapore, Panasonic opened a fully automated indoor farm for 81 tons of vegetables every year. Aero Farms in Newark, USA, opened the largest so far, a nine-meter-high warehouse that will supply 250 different unsprayed vegetables and herbs.

Greenhouses are an area where machines are still surprisingly absent: picking crops such as tomatoes, peppers and strawberries has not yet been spent on robot hands on a large scale. Throughout the year, armies of pickers move into the greenhouses, which usually have relatively low wages and long and arduous working days. The picking robot is already used in Japan. In the absence of cheap labour, farmers there are in some cases satisfied with robots that harvest far less than human pickers. Even if the robot only harvests sixty or seventy percent of all strawberries, the grower earns more than if he hires relatively expensive pickers.

Agriculture on saline soils

- On Texel they succeeded in growing potatoes and vegetables on saline ground.
- Worldwide, 1.5 billion hectares of agricultural land are threatened by salinization. In areas where salinization poses the greatest threat, this offers a chance to feed families independently.
- Can the salty potato save people from the famine? Since 2010, Zilt Proefbedrijf Texel has been researching which crops grow on salty soil. Many species do well.
- The fermentation of seaweed releases 2/3 methane gas and 1/3 hydrogen gas which must only be collected and used better than the alternatives for natural gas that are currently available.

Sexual freedom

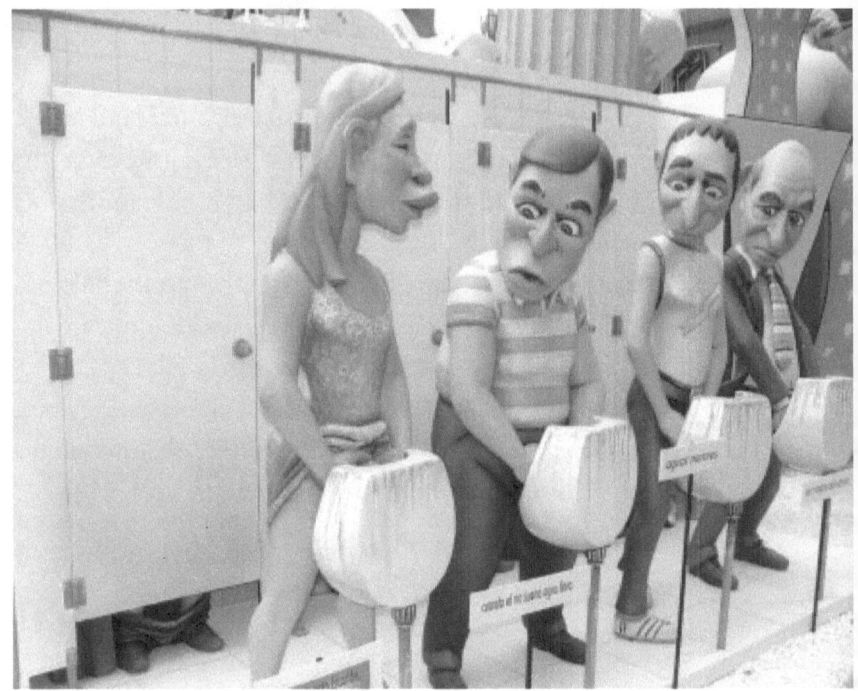

The first transgender was spotted in Alicante, 2018

The discovery of the pill was a great revolution. For the first time in human history, sexual intercourse and reproduction could be technically and artificially separated. The enormous commercial success was blinding, both for medicine and for theology. And everyone tried to outdo the other in giving good justification for birth control. Contraception caused a radical break with the lives of all previous generations and civilizations. Legal abortion has since been introduced, the number of divorces has increased spectacularly, euthanasia has been advocated if life is no longer experienced as meaningful. The family as the basis of church and society has crumbled into all sorts of free living together. All forms of sexuality are then openly discussed. The emergence of gays, Me Too for unwanted intimacies, sexual intimidation and rape, incest and pedophilia, gender change of transgender people, genital mutilation in other cultures. The sexual abstinence from celibacy also had its problems such as pedophilia in priests.

Yet the balance of sudden sexual freedom is positive overall, thanks to the increased emancipation of women and the awareness of sexual problems and liberties that have been hidden for years. There are more and more women in managerial positions. There have been Queens for quite some time, but now women have also become ministers and president. We are still waiting for the first woman as pope, now that the woman has also been admitted to church.

In the metropolis of Ghuangzhou (the former Canton), our guide pointed us to a female Buddha in the largest temple.

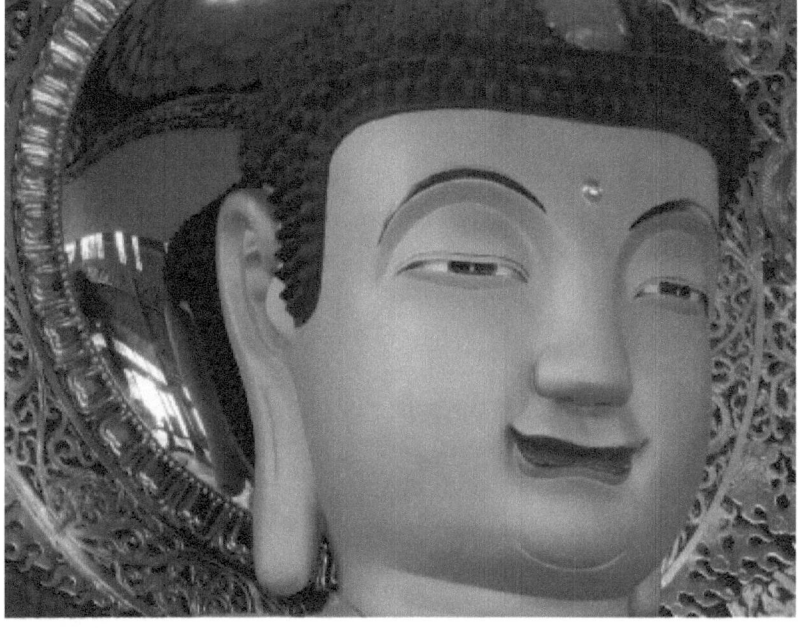

The orgasm has a protective effect on health

Evolution of spontaneous ovulation in mammals is correlated with increasing distance from the clitoris to the copulatory canal. With the evolution of spontaneous ovulation, the female orgasm was freed to gain secondary roles. which may explain its maintenance. Regular brushing your teeth is just as important as a regular orgasm. At least one to three times a day's brushing is required. *Keep smiling until you have no more teeth.* An orgasm one to three times a month is needed to prevent aging processes and to stay healthy. Our famous and charming Flemish sexologist Goedele Liekens has already indicated that she may come to her convenience without penetrating sex and without steady relationship with a man.

Half of the women over 80 always or almost always reach the state of sexual satisfaction. Although frequency of arousal, lubrication, and orgasm decreased with age, the youngest (<55 years) **and** oldest (>80 years) women reported a higher frequency of orgasm satisfaction. This is according to a study among 806 women in and around San Diego in the US, published in the American Journal of Medicine.

Trompeter SE, Bettencourt R, Barrett-Connor E Sexual activity and satisfaction in healthy community-dwelling older women. Am J Med. 2012 Jan; 125 (1): 37-43
https://www.ncbi.nlm.nih.gov/pubmed/22195529

Evidence suggests that ejaculation frequency may be inversely related to the risk of prostate cancer (PCa), a disease for which few modifiable risk factors have been identified.

Rider JR, Wilson KM, Sinnott JA et al. Ejaculation Frequency and Risk of Prostate Cancer: Updated Results with an Additional Decade of Follow-up.
Euro Urol. 2016 Dec;70(6):947-982

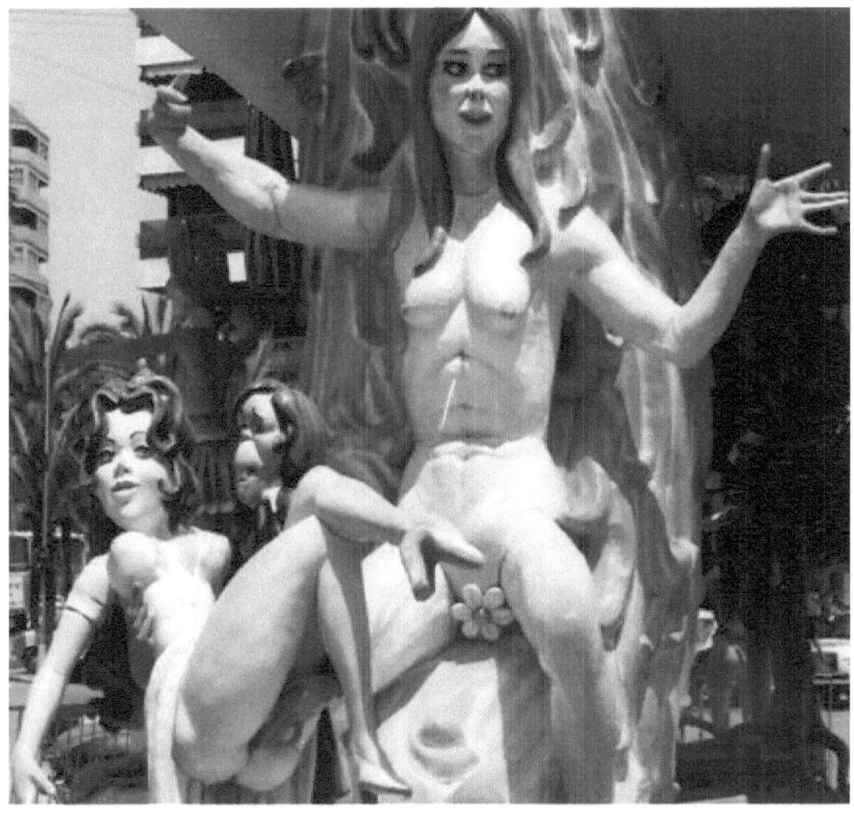

Happy company, rubbing makes it itchy and itching makes you rub

Men who have two orgasms or more per week are half as likely to die than other men.

Davey Smith G[1][1], Frankel S[2], Yarnell J[3]. Sex and death: are they related? Findings from the Caerphilly Cohort Study. BMJ.[4] 1997 Dec 20-27;315(7123):1641-4.

Mortality risk was 50% lower in the group with high orgasmic frequency than in the group with low orgasmic frequency. Death from coronary heart disease and from other causes showed similar associations with frequency of orgasm, although the gradient was most marked for deaths from coronary heart disease.

What is the function of orgasm?

In the earliest animal species the hormones released during orgasm induced ovulation. In these very first mammals, ovulation is triggered by sexual penetration. In 2016, the Pavlicev team analyzed 41 species of mammals. Refelex ovulation occurs in 15 of these species, including cats, koalas, rabbits and camels. Mammals appear to be the first in which generation of ovulation has evolved. With 75 million years, spontaneous ovulation (and thus the menstrual cycle) is a recent development in the evolution of life on earth.

Human female orgasm is associated with an endocrine surge similar to the copulatory surges in species with induced ovulation. Evolution of spontaneous ovulation in mammals is correlated with increasing distance from the clitoris to the copulatory canal. With the evolution of spontaneous ovulation, orgasm was freed to gain secondary roles. which may explain its maintenance.

In an orgasm, the brain releases several hormones or signal substances.

---

1.   https://www.ncbi.nlm.nih.gov/

        pubmed/?term=Davey%20Smith%20G%5BAuthor%5D&cauthor=true&cauthor_uid=9448525

2.   https://www.ncbi.nlm.nih.gov/

        pubmed/?term=Frankel%20S%5BAuthor%5D&cauthor=true&cauthor_uid=9448525

3.   https://www.ncbi.nlm.nih.gov/

        pubmed/?term=Yarnell%20J%5BAuthor%5D&cauthor=true&cauthor_uid=9448525

4.   https://www.ncbi.nlm.nih.gov/pubmed/9448525

- **Dopamine.** With an orgasm release brain cells from the substantia negra dopamine. The substantia nigra, or black core, is a pigment-containing core in the mesencephalon, or the middle part of the brain. The basal nuclei and the black nuclei (substantia nigra) in the brain play a very important role in making movements run smoothly.

In Parkinson's disease, a deficiency of the neurotransmitter dopamine occurs in the brain. Cells that produce dopamine die slowly. These cells are mainly located in the substantia nigra. In Parkinson's disease the basal ganglia no longer receives dopamine from the substantia nigra, which means that the patient can move less and less well.

- **Oxytocine.** Through the orgasm, the brain also injects the hormone oxytocin into the body - a hormone that promotes muscle contractions around the genitals and ejaculation.
- **Vasopressine.** Brain scans show that the left orbito-frontal lobe has less blood circulation during orgasm than during a state of high sexual arousal without orgasm. "We know that this area is involved in controlling all kinds of drives," says neuroanatoma Janniko Georgiadis. "This is also known from psychopathology. An example is that of Phineas Gage, an American railway worker from the 19th century who received an iron bar through his skull at this location. He survived the accident, but afterwards was enormously sexually disinhibited. "Other areas of the brain are extra active. This applies, for example, to the small brain. These are probably involved in muscle contractions that are typical of orgasm. The researcher also found a connection between the degree of sexual arousal and the blood circulation in the middle brain. There are dopamine producing cells. This may mean that dopamine plays a role in sexual arousal during orgasm.

- **Endorphin.** Endorphin, also called the lucky hormone, is a neurotransmitter. Neurotransmitters are messengers of your brain and give stimuli from one nerve cell to another. Endorphins make you less sensitive to pain. In addition to suppressing pain, it also increases resistance, provides a feeling of happiness and reduces anxiety. It strongly resembles morphine.

References

The National Center for Biotechnology Information (NCBI) was established in 1988 as a department of the National Institutes of Health. NIH was selected for their experience in creating and maintaining bio-medical databases. The collection of research reports from NIH represent the largest biomedical research facility in the world.

All the studies mentioned in this book can be consulted on the internet page of the NCBI by entering the matching database number.

For example: Is breast cancer a zoonosis?

Szabo S, Haislip AM, Garry RF (2005) Of mice, cats, and men: is human breast cancer a zoonosis? Microsc Res Tech. 68(3-4):197-208. Review

https://www.ncbi.nlm.nih.gov/pubmed/16276516

Malignant lymphomas and Chlamydia pneumoniae infections

Chronic infections can predict malignant growth. A connection has been shown of chronic Chlamydia pneumoniae infection with lung cancer. In the study of Anttila TI an association was found between chronic C. pneumoniae infections and malignant lymphomas (Anttila TI). The link was most present with Non-Hodgkin lymphoma (OR = 7.3, 95% CI 2.2 to 25).25)

Healing of malignant lymphoma with doxycycline

Chlamydia psittaci (Cp), the bacterium of psittacose has often been shown in malignant lymphomas. The bacterium has been shown in the tumor tissue, taken out and cell cultures are made. By treatment with doxycycline malignant lymphomas are cured (Ferreri AJ).

Ferreri AJ, Dolcetti R, Magnino S ey al. (2007) A woman and her canary: a tale of chlamydiae and lymphomas. J Natl Cancer Inst. 2007 Sep 19;99(18):1418-9
https://www.ncbi.nlm.nih.gov/pubmed/17848672

Treatment with doxycycline (twice daily 100 mg) for six months disappeared the malignant lymphomas in 64% of patients. Tetracycline and macrolide (erythromycin) antibiotics have a remarkable therapeutic effect on Cp infection. Cp infection is thus controllable.

Chlamydiae have no cell wall and, like viruses, are completely dependent on their host cells. Once in the host cell, Chlamydiae is not sensitive to penicillin. Tetracycline enters cells in the contaminated body cells by diffusion along membrane pores. Once in the cell, tetracyclines and doxycycline inhibit internal cell metabolism, DNA and protein synthesis, whereby Chlamydia cell parasites cannot create new proteins for growth and proliferation.

Anttila TI, Lehtinen T, Leinonen M, Bloigu A, Koskela P, Lehtinen M, Saikku P (1998) Serological evidence of an association between chlamydial infections and malignant lymphomas. Br J Haematol. Oct;103(1):150-6.

https://www.ncbi.nlm.nih.gov/pubmed/9792302

Ferreri AJ 2005, Ponzoni M, Guidoboni M et al. Regression of ocular adnexal lymphoma after Chlamydia psittaci-eradicating antibiotic therapy. J Clin Oncol 2005, 23:5067–5073.

Ferreri AJ, Ponzoni M, Guidoboni M et al. (2006) Bacteria-eradicating therapy with doxycycline in ocular adnexal MALT lymphoma: a multicenter prospective trial. J Natl Cancer Inst 98:1375– 1382.

https://www.ncbi.nlm.nih.gov/pubmed/15968003

Ferreri AJ, Govi S, Pasini E et al. (2012) Chlamydophila Psittaci Eradication with Doxycycline as first-line targeted therapy for Ocular Adnexae Lymphoma: Final Results of International Phase II Trial. J Clin Oncol 3

https://www.ncbi.nlm.nih.gov/pubmed/22802315

Autobiography

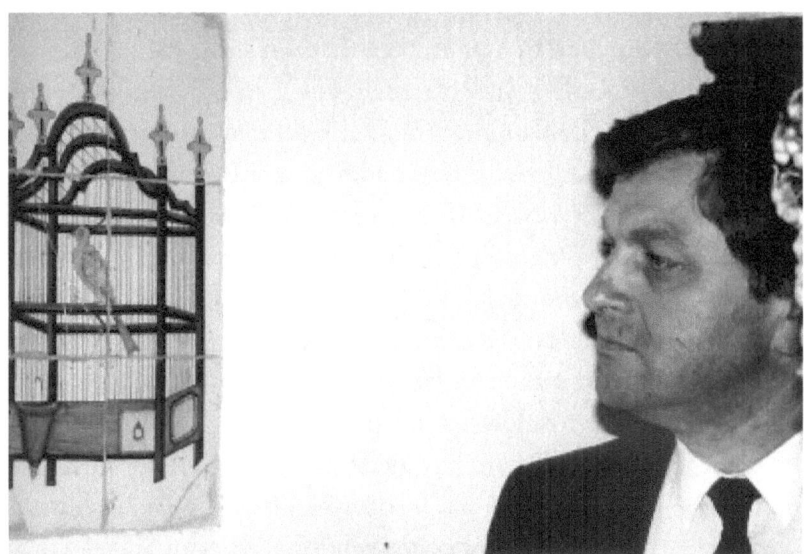

Peter Holst was born on Sunday 10 October 1943 during the church service in Sint Philipsland on the island of Tholen in Zeeland. His father Pelgrim Holst was the predecessor and was standing in the pulpit at that time. The sexton who normally brought a glass of water to the pulpit now came up with the message "the delivery went well, and it is a boy". His father was a minister at the Dutch Reformed congregation and the church service that lasted at least one hour was normally ended. Pastor Pelgrim Holst has about 1,000 marriages consecrated to the church with the promise of eternal loyalty. He was a very successful pastor.

Peter A.J. Holst went to study health care at the University of Utrecht. At this university, lectures and practice were combined at the faculties of human medicine, veterinary medicine and dentistry until the candidate exam. For his bachelor he did his pathology exam with Professor A. de Minjer. His thesis on small cell lung cancer was discussed and the Minjer took him to the pottery museum where they

145

stopped for some time in front of a preparation with lung carcinoma of a smoker. De Minjer pointed out to him that lung cancer and breast cancer for the coming years would be the biggest challenges of medicine. More than fifty years later, that is still the case.

After assistantships in Rotterdam and Leiden, he graduated from the University of Leiden in 1969. During the midwifery internship in Leiden, Professor A. Sikkel asked him to assist in the practice of Dr. P.J. Meijst in Hazerswoude. In the event of a collision on the provincial road, this general practitioner had broken his shoulder and had to be assisted for several months in the practice. An additional advantage was that during this period there would certainly be some deliveries where I could assist. That came true because during my assistantship I could lead more home deliveries than I could have done in the obstetric clinic in Leiden. Professor Sikkel has made contraception an indispensable part of the profession and, has institutionalized the establishment of a separate outpatient clinic for contraception. Professor Sikkel was a very inspiring doctor.

Holst worked as a general practitioner in Rijswijk-Den Haag from 1970 to 1984. In his early years as a general practitioner, Holst was also supervisor of a clinic for birth control in Delft (Dr. Rutgers Foundation) for several years. The Rutgers Foundation was successful in the seventies of the twentieth century with its counseling agencies for contraception, the Rutgershuizen. In 1969 and 1970 he held evening consultation hours at the Rutgershuis in Delft. Dr. J. Karbaat, then director of the Zuiderziekenhuis in Rotterdam, also held consultation hours at this office and taught him to place IUDs. When the St Hippolytus hospital on the Phoenixstraat in Delft moved to a new location, the former hospital was transformed into a business collection building. Under the direction of Holst, the incubator department on the top floor of this building was converted into a number of consultation and examination rooms of the new Rutgershuis in Delft. He has placed about 250 IUDs in all of the following practical years, including in his own general practice during evening consultation hours for contraception and cervical smears. He held back-guard consultation hours for the morning after pill. Real 'Hagueneses' then asked for the **"morning after save pill"**.

Under influence of the Nederlands Huisartsen Instituut, his practice was set up from the beginning with a surveillance schedule. This means that age groups are always tested for the risks that occur in the age group. As additional operations during consultation contacts at least once the blood pressure was measured, for example also once from 50 years the eye pressure measured and noted, the stool examined for occult blood loss from 50 years, in risk groups also an electrocardiogram was made, etc. At the beginning of my general practice, I found a severe pneumonia in a young woman of 20 years old. After treatment with an antibiotic she recovered. Because she had a cage with a parakeet in her bedroom, I wondered whether the presence of a cage bird in the house could possibly cause more serious illness. A 17 years old boy died of bone cancer in his leg during the first years of my practice. This young man had constantly kept and bred at least 100 tropical songbirds in a basement. One can imagine the risk of repeated bird flu and the occurrence of blood and bone marrow episodes with slow-moving carcinogenic bone infection in such intensive contact. Because of the many consultation hours and home visits, ten lung cancer patients came to my attention in a year. Of these, there were six bird keepers in the years before diagnosis. After consulting with professor F. de Waard of the RIVM, department of epidemiology, I have set up a ten-year practice survey and follow-up studies. The statistical link was demonstrated, later confirmed in studies in Berlin and Glasgow. Much later, in 2012 a laboratory experiment proved the link between lung cancer and Chlamydia pneumonia infection.

In 1987, this research led to his PhD at the University of Utrecht on the relationship he demonstrated between breeding and keeping birds indoors and lung cancer. He defended the hypothesis that lung cancer in bird keepers and bird breeders is the result of persistent infection of the deeper basal cells in the airways. These basal cells are still multipotent and do not die if the cell is infected with a bacterium like the Chlamydia that can only propagate in a living host cell. His promoters were prof. F. de Waard, epidemiologist of the RIVM, professor P. Zwart, special veterinary faculty and D. Kromhout, nutritional epidemiologist.

The practical studies and the dust measurements with TNO were supported by the Dutch Prevention Fund. After this he started working as director of Health, Safety and Environment services.

After his retirement in 2005, he started traveling a lot. Born in Zeeland (1943), on land in the sea, the sea-hole and the wide world continued to attract him. He has crossed all the oceans several times after more than 20 cruises. The volcanic islands in the Pacific Ocean are very impressive. All first life forms originated here and spread out from South America to Africa, Europe, Asia and Australia. From the primordial soup of the Pacific Ocean the fish, amphibians, birds, dinosaurs and mammals originated. From around 4,000 years ago, the 10,000 Polynesian islands in the Pacific Ocean were populated by the Chinese from Taiwan and South-East China. The oldest cultures are found in the Far East.

Very special, in North and South America there are no great apes, only howler monkeys and capuchin monkeys. The great apes and homo sapiens have arisen in central Africa.

Holst has had his own practice for 14 years and then worked for 20 years as a specialist in working conditions, lifestyle, indoor air and environmental factors. His interest in the link between breeding tropical birds and cancer has expanded to the health risks of the intensive rearing of poultry, pigs and cattle for consumption. Since the fifties of the 20th century, intensive breeding in livestock has increased sharply. An increase that keeps pace with the recent increase in cancer mortality.

More books from the author

Auteur: Peter A.J. Holst MD PhD

Pet birds and hazards to health, 1987. Eburon ISBN 90-70879-76-X Delft

Birdkeeping as a Source of Lung Cancer and Other Human Diseases. A Need for Higher Hygienic Standards, 1991
Springer-Verlag ISBN 3-540- 53555-1, Berlin/Heidelberg
Springer-Verlag ISBN 3-387-53555-1, New York

Caged birds and laying hens can cause cancer in man. 2013
E-book APPLE ISBN 978-90-818776-7-1
Paperback ISBN 978-94-021119-0-02

The Last Chimpanzee, somewhere in the 21st century, the last chimpanzee will die. 2014
E-book APPLE
Paperback ISBN 978-94-02124-8-4

Plant-Based food is your Best Medicine. 2015
E-book APPLE 106 pages ISBN 9789082210569

Vegetarian Food everyday keeps your doctor away. 2016
E-book APPLE 144 pages

Common Cancers are Zoonoses. 2016
E-book APPLE 197 pages ISBN 978-90-824963-3-8

Increase in Cancer is a Recent Event. 2016
E-book Apple ISBN 978-90-824963-0-7

PREVENTION IS BETTER THAN CURE. 2016
E-book 978-90-824963-2-1

The Blueprint of Cancer, how to change your lifestyle and eating habits. 2016 e-book 234 pages ISBN 978-90-822105-9-0

Stop the Meatballs. 2019
Paperback 131 pages ISBN 978-1797658926

Our Inheritance from the Great Apes. 2019
Paperback. 146 pages ISBN 978-1081342159

Canimalism. 2019
E-book Kindle 119 pages
Paperback 120 pages Amazon.com ISBN 978-1694357762
Hardcover 120 pages Bravenewbooks.nl ISBN 978-9402198577

Specification of writing and photos

Prior to the invention of the art of printing, texts were multiplied by copying them manually. In the Middle Ages, monks occupied themselves with manual "copying" of books for months on end. The invention of the letterpress in the 15th century unleashed a revolution in the dissemination of knowledge and ideas.

Self publishing has become possible since the beginning of the 21st century. You can publish a manuscript in a Word document as an ebook via draft2digital.com. The ebook is also available on Kobo, iBooks and Bol.com. The paperback can be created from a pdf document at Amazon.com via KDP. The hardcover can finally be published via Bravenewbooks. and will be placed on Bol.com.

Photos